T0206073

SpringerBriefs in Statistics

JSS Research Series in Statistics

Editors-in-Chief

Naoto Kunitomo
Akimichi Takemura

Series editors

Genshiro Kitagawa
Tomoyuki Higuchi
Yutaka Kano
Toshimitsu Hamasaki
Shigeyuki Matsui
Manabu Iwasaki
Yasuhiro Omori
Masafumi Akahira

The current research of statistics in Japan has expanded in several directions in line with recent trends in academic activities in the area of statistics and statistical sciences over the globe. The core of these research activities in statistics in Japan has been the Japan Statistical Society (JSS). This society, the oldest and largest academic organization for statistics in Japan, was founded in 1931 by a handful of pioneer statisticians and economists and now has a history of about 80 years. Many distinguished scholars have been members, including the influential statistician Hirotugu Akaike, who was a past president of JSS, and the notable mathematician Kiyosi Itô, who was an earlier member of the Institute of Statistical Mathematics (ISM), which has been a closely related organization since the establishment of ISM. The society has two academic journals: the Journal of the Japan Statistical Society (English Series) and the Journal of the Japan Statistical Society (Japanese Series). The membership of JSS consists of researchers, teachers, and professional statisticians in many different fields including mathematics, statistics, engineering, medical sciences, government statistics, economics, business, psychology, education, and many other natural, biological, and social sciences.

The JSS Series of Statistics aims to publish recent results of current research activities in the areas of statistics and statistical sciences in Japan that otherwise would not be available in English; they are complementary to the two JSS academic journals, both English and Japanese. Because the scope of a research paper in academic journals inevitably has become narrowly focused and condensed in recent years, this series is intended to fill the gap between academic research activities and the form of a single academic paper.

The series will be of great interest to a wide audience of researchers, teachers, professional statisticians, and graduate students in many countries who are interested in statistics and statistical sciences, in statistical theory, and in various areas of statistical applications.

More information about this series at http://www.springer.com/series/13497

Takeshi Emura · Yi-Hau Chen

Analysis of Survival Data with Dependent Censoring

Copula-Based Approaches

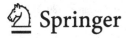
Springer

Takeshi Emura
Graduate Institute of Statistics
National Central University
Taoyuan
Taiwan

Yi-Hau Chen
Institute of Statistical Science
Academia Sinica
Taipei
Taiwan

ISSN 2191-544X   ISSN 2191-5458   (electronic)
SpringerBriefs in Statistics
ISSN 2364-0057   ISSN 2364-0065   (electronic)
JSS Research Series in Statistics
ISBN 978-981-10-7163-8   ISBN 978-981-10-7164-5   (eBook)
https://doi.org/10.1007/978-981-10-7164-5

Library of Congress Control Number: 2017964253

Printed on acid-free paper

This Springer imprint is published by the registered company Springer Nature Singapore Pte Ltd. part of Springer Nature
The registered company address is: 152 Beach Road, #21-01/04 Gateway East, Singapore 189721, Singapore

Preface

About this Book

This book introduces copula-based statistical methods to analyze survival data involving dependent censoring. This book explains why the problem of dependent censoring arises in medical research, and illustrates how copula-based statistical methods remedy the problem. This book introduces a variety of copula-based methods to deal with dependent censoring, including the copula-graphic estimator, parametric/semi-parametric maximum likelihood estimators, univariate selection method, and prediction method. This book also introduces the basic theory of copulas for modeling bivariate survival data.

There are many general books on survival analysis such as Kalbfleisch and Prentice (2002), Lawless (2003), Klein and Moeschberger (2003), and Collett (2003, 2015). These books focus on the standard statistical methods that have been developed under the assumption of independent censoring. Nonetheless, all these books mention the importance of scrutinizing the independent censoring assumption when applying the standard methods to real data. Kalbfleisch and Prentice (2002), Lawless (2003), and Klein and Moeschberger (2003) provide competing risks approaches to deal with dependent censoring without using copulas. In his latest edition of "Modelling Survival Data in Medical Research," Collett (2015) added a new chapter, "Dependent Censoring," where some techniques of dealing with dependent censoring are introduced. Our book introduces a variety of copula-based statistical methods that are not discussed in the above-listed books.

Our emphasis is placed on survival data arising from medical studies. I hope that this book appeals to those working as (bio) statisticians in medical and pharmaceutical institutes. Of course, statistical methods presented in this book can be applied to many fields, especially in engineering and econometrics where survival analysis plays an important role.

Use as a Textbook

Readers (instructors) may begin with the basic survival analysis in Chap. 2 and then proceed gradually to study advanced topics in Chaps. 3–5. This book may be used as a textbook for classroom teaching aimed at graduate students or a short course aimed at (bio) statisticians.

Alternatively, readers may study each chapter independently. Perhaps, students majoring in science or rigorous statisticians may feel comfortable to read Chaps. 2 and 3 before Chaps. 4 and 5. On the other hand, biostatisticians who have learned to use survival analysis may directly start from Chap. 5; they might be more interested in how to implement the new methods with R and how to interpret the outputs. Chapter 6 collects open problems for future research. This might help find research topics for students and researchers.

Exercises are attached to Chaps. 2 and 3, though readers are certainly not necessary to complete them. Nevertheless, ambitious readers or students seeking their thesis topics are encouraged to work on them.

Taoyuan, Taiwan   Takeshi Emura
Taipei, Taiwan   Yi-Hau Chen

References

Collett D (2003) Modelling survival data in medical research, 2nd edn. CRC press, London
Collett D (2015) Modelling survival data in medical research, 3rd edn. CRC press, London
Kalb fleisch JD, Prentice RL (2002) The statistical analysis of failure time data, 2nd edn. Wiley, New York
Klein JP, Moeschberger ML (2003) Survival analysis techniques for censored and truncated data. Springer, New York
Lawless JF (2003) Statistical models and methods for lifetime data, 2nd edn. Wiley, New Jersey

Acknowledgements

We thank the series editor, Dr. Toshimitsu Hamasaki, for his invitation to write this book and his valuable suggestions on this book. We also thank Mr. Jia-Han Shih for his comments and suggestions on this book and his effort for checking the solutions to the exercises (the solution manual may be available from Shih J-H). We also thank Ms. Sayaka Shinohara for working on some formulas in Appendix A. Emura T and Chen YH are financially supported by Ministry of Science and Technology, Taiwan (MOST 105-2118-M-008-003-MY2; MOST 104-2118-M-001-006-MY3).

Contents

Abbreviations

CG estimator	Copula-graphic estimator
FGM copula	Farlie–Gumbel–Morgenstern copula
MLE	Maximum likelihood estimator
OS	Overall survival
PI	Prognostic index
RR	Relative risk
SD	Standard deviation
SE	Standard error

Notations

$a \in A$	An element a belonging to a set A
$\mathbf{a}'$	The transpose of a column vector $\mathbf{a}$
$E[X\,|Y]$	The conditional expectation of X given Y
$f : A \mapsto B$	A function from the domain A to the range B
$\frac{f(t+dt)}{dt}$	The limit of $\frac{f(t+\Delta t)}{\Delta t}$ as $\Delta t \to 0$
$N(0, 1)$	The standard normal distribution
$\mathbf{I}(\,\cdot\,)$	The indicator function: $\mathbf{I}(A) = 1$ if A is true, or $\mathbf{I}(A) = 0$ if A is false
$\Pr(A|B)$	The conditional probability of A given B

Chapter 1
Setting the Scene

Abstract This first chapter presents the purpose of the book. We first illustrate the issues of dependent censoring arising from medical research. We then explain several benefits of investigating dependent censoring. We finally illustrate how copula-based methods have been grown through the literature of survival analysis.

Keywords Censoring · Competing risk · Cox regression · Endpoint
Informative dropout · Multivariate survival analysis · Overall survival

1.1 Survival Analysis and Censoring

Survival analysis is a branch of statistics concerned with event times. In many examples of survival analysis, event times may be time-to-death as the name *survival* suggests. Time-to-death for patients is termed *overall survival* (OS) which is considered as the most objective measure of patient health in cancer research.

Analysis of survival data is complicated by *censoring*. If patient follow-up is terminated before observing time-to-death, they are said to be *censored*. Censoring is unavoidable in survival data; the study has a planned end of follow-up, or patients may decide to withdraw from the study. Typically, medical researchers and statisticians analyze survival data by assuming that censoring mechanisms are unrelated to the event of interest. Indeed, standard tools in survival analysis, such as the Kaplan–Meier estimator and Cox regression, deal with censoring under the assumption that event time and censoring time are statistically independent.

If censoring mechanisms involve dropout or withdrawal due to a worsening of the symptoms, censoring may introduce bias into the results of statistical analysis. This type of dropout is often called *informative dropout*. Informative dropout is just one of many contributing causes of censoring. More generally, if event time of interest is censored by any mechanism related to the event, this phenomenon shall be referred to *dependent censoring*. Most of the standard survival analysis methods give unbiased results under the *independent censoring assumption*; that is, censoring mechanisms are unrelated to the event of interest.

© The Author(s) 2018
T. Emura and Y.-H. Chen, *Analysis of Survival Data with Dependent Censoring*,
JSS Research Series in Statistics, https://doi.org/10.1007/978-981-10-7164-5_1

The book hopes to provide a systematic account of the issues of dependent censoring and to give survival analysis methods that apply *copulas* to appropriately deal with the issues.

1.2 Informative Dropout

In a medical follow-up study for cancer patients, survival time may be censored at the time of dropout owing to tumor progression, toxicity of treatment, initiation of second treatment, etc. Then, overall survival and dropout time may be positively correlated because a patient may typically die soon after dropout. This leads to informative dropout. Some discussions about the issues of informative dropout and dependent censoring are found in Kalbfleish and Prentice (2002), Chen (2010), Staplin (2012), Collett (2015), Staplin et al. (2015), Emura and Chen (2016), and references therein.

Censoring due to informative dropout may have a deleterious effect on the results of data analysis. Consider a case, where many terminally ill patients have dropped out of a clinical trial to stay in the comfort of their own home. This means that the data collected on the clinical trial miss many deaths that could be observed. Consequently, the Kaplan–Meier survival curve that treats those patients as censoring (i.e., being alive at their dropout) may exhibit upward bias. The Cox regression analysis can adjust the bias if there are covariates that can predict the occurrence of dropout and other causes of censoring.

Dependent censoring refers to the situation where the dependence between censoring time and survival time is not explained by observable covariates. In other words, dependent censoring is a consequence of residual dependence that is not adjusted by covariates. In a sense, the concern for dependent censoring is reduced by collecting as many covariates as possible. For instance, a late-stage cancer patient may result in short survival and high chance to drop out due to tumor progression, which gives the positive dependence between survival and dropout times. Hence, the cancer stage can be included as one of covariates to achieve the conditional independence between survival and dropout. Some diagnostic plots are suggested to detect residual dependence (Chap. 14 of Collett (2015); Siannis et al. 2005; Chap. 5 of this book).

Residual dependence causes the partial likelihood estimator (Cox 1972) to be biased. Suppose that one wishes to assess the effect of a covariate x_1 on overall survival through the Cox model $h(t|x_1) = h_0(t) \exp(\beta_1 x_1)$, where β_1 represents the covariate effect and $h_0(t)$ is the baseline hazard function. The partial likelihood estimator gives a consistent estimate for β_1 under the conditional independence assumption between overall survival and censoring time given x_1. Unfortunately, if there exists another covariate x_2 influencing both survival and dropout, the conditional independence assumption would be violated as the variation of x_2 induces residual dependence (Fig. 1.1).

Fig. 1.1 A mechanism of yielding residual dependence between survival and dropout triggered by an unmeasured covariate

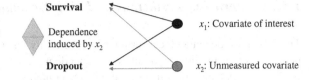

Indeed, the so-called shared frailty models are derived as a consequence of residual dependence due to unmeasured covariates (Oakes 1989). While the frailty models are not the main focus of this book, they are helpful to introduce a mechanism of residual dependence. In Chap. 3, we shall provide more systematic discussions about residual dependence by relating the shared frailty models with the copula models.

1.3 Benefits of Investigating Dependent Censoring

As mentioned earlier, a motivation to study dependent censoring emerges from medical research. Researchers may demand a bivariate survival model to specify the interrelationship between survival time and censoring time. This book introduces copulas as the main tool for constructing such models. In the following, we shall pick up specific advantages for adopting copula-based approaches to deal with dependent censoring.

1.3.1 Examining the Influence of Dependent Censoring

If researchers perform the Cox regression analysis by incorrectly imposing the independent censoring assumption, estimates of regression coefficients can be biased. Emura and Chen (2016) applied copulas to examine the bias owing to residual dependence. These analyses show that the bias is influenced by the rate of censoring, the degree of dependence, and the type of copulas. This issue shall be detailed in Chap. 3. Beside this method, copulas provide a variety of sensitivity analyses. The copula-graphic estimator (Zheng and Klein 1995; Rivest and Wells 2001) can be used to examine how the survival curve is influenced by dependent censoring. Likelihood-based sensitivity analyses are referred to Chen (2010) under a semi-parametric model and Emura and Michimae (2017) under a parametric model. Moradian et al. (2017) applied copulas to see the influence of dependence on survival forests. Sugimoto et al. (2017) adopted copula models to examine the influence of dependent censoring on the power and sample size of the log-rank test in clinical trials with multiple endpoints.

1.3.2 Improving Prediction by Using Dependent Censoring

The effect of dependent censoring can potentially be useful for improving the performance of prediction. Intuitively, dependent censoring due to patient dropout is related to patients' health status and hence contains some predictive information about OS. Siannis et al. (2005) proposed a graphical diagnostic method by plotting a *prognostic index* against a *censoring index* (see also Chap. 14 of Collett 2015). If the censoring index is positively correlated with the prognostic index, high risk of death is predicted by high intensity of censoring.

The diagnostic procedure has a certain drawback that requires parametric models to be fitted to both OS and censoring time. This strong assumption is understandable due to the identifiability problem of the competing risks relationship between OS and censoring time. Indeed, developing prediction models is a challenging problem. Chapter 5 is devoted to the idea of Emura and Chen (2016) who proposed an alternative diagnostic plot and a prediction method for OS by utilizing the information of dependent censoring.

1.4 Copulas and Survival Analysis: A Brief History

Briefly speaking, a copula is a function to link two random variables by specifying their dependence structure. A mathematician, Abe Sklar, first used the word copula in his study of probabilistic metric space (Sklar 1959). In his paper, he gave a mathematical definition of copulas and established the most fundamental theorem about copulas, known as Sklar's theorem. More about copulas can be found in the book of Nelsen (2006).

Apparently, the applications of copulas in survival analysis became active after David George Clayton introduced his bivariate survival model (Clayton 1978). David Oakes soon realized the importance of Clayton's model and reformulated Clayton's bivariate survival model into its current form (Oakes 1982). While neither Clayton nor Oakes mentioned about copulas, their work yielded one of the most important copulas for bivariate survival analysis, later known as *the Clayton copula*.

Clayton's model is regarded as the *gamma frailty model*, a special case of *shared frailty models* (Oakes 1989). On the other hand, Clayton's model is a special case of *Archimedean copula* models (Genest and MacKay 1986). Oakes (1989) touched upon the paper of Genest and Mackay (1986) but did not mention about copulas. Many important works on bivariate survival analysis were generated under Clayton's model without mentioning about Archimedean copulas. These include the estimation procedure of Hsu and Prentice (1996) and the goodness-of-fit test of Shih (1998).

One of the earliest papers that successfully and explicitly applied copulas to the bivariate survival data seems to be Shih and Louis (1995) who proposed a two-stage estimation approach. They used copulas to develop a unified estimation method applicable to many copulas, rather than the method specific to Clayton's model. See also Burzykowski et al. (2001, 2005) for studying the association between survival endpoints based on copulas. Later on, the goodness-of-fit test of Shih (1998) that was developed solely for Clayton's model was generalized to a unified test applicable to a broad class of bivariate survival models described by Archimedean copulas (Emura et al. 2010).

While the method of Shih and Louis (1995) can handle bivariate event times, it essentially requires the assumption of independent censorship. An inconvenience occurs if one event time censors the other. For instance, death dependently censors time-to-tumor progression. Hence, it is not a valid way to apply the two-stage estimation by treating time-to-tumor progression and overall survival as bivariate event times subject to independent censoring. This problem is known as *competing risks* or *dependent censoring*. In general, estimation with competing risks data is substantially more challenging than estimation with bivariate survival data due to the identifiability issue (Tsiatis 1975); competing risks data do not allow one to observe two event times simultaneously (one event censors the other), and hence, the data may not identify the dependence structure between event times.

The paper by Zheng and Klein (1995) gave a partial solution to the identifiability problem of dependent censoring by an *assumed copula* between two event times. They generalized the Kaplan–Meier estimator under independent censoring to the *copula-graphic (CG) estimator* under dependent censoring. For Archimedean copula models, Rivest and Wells (2001) obtained the explicit expression of the CG estimator, derived its asymptotic properties using a martingale theory, and formulated a sensitivity analysis on the choice of the assumed copula. Nowadays, the CG estimator is one of the most important tools for analyzing data with competing risks or dependent censoring (Staplin 2012; de Uña-Álvarez and Veraverbeke 2013, 2017; Emura and Chen 2016; Emura and Michimae 2017; Moradian et al. 2017). Note that the CG estimator is still of limited use for fitting real medical data since it cannot handle covariates.

Braekers and Veraverbeke (2005) extended the CG estimator to deal with a covariate. Unfortunately, this approach is too restrictive in medical applications since it cannot handle more than one covariate. Indeed, all the CG-type estimators are derived from moment-based equations, which may not be naturally extended to handle covariates.

Likelihood-based approaches can naturally deal with covariates under an assumed copula for dependent censoring. Likelihood-based regression analyses are straightforward and workable under parametric models (Escarela and Carrière 2003), though the full parametric assumptions are too strong in many medical applications. Alternatively, Chen (2010) adopted a semi-parametric likelihood method to perform regression under bivariate competing risks models, where the copula is assumed and the marginal distributions follow the transformation Cox model. Chen's method reduces to the partial likelihood method under the independence copula and the identity transformation.

The copula-based approaches are further extended to handle *semi-competing risks* data. Fine et al. (2001) introduced the concept of semi-competing risks in which a non-terminal event can be censored by a terminal event, but not vice versa. This brings an alternative solution to the identifiability of a model of dependent censoring by removing the competing risk for the terminal event time. Their statistical approach was developed under Clayton's model, and it was later extended to Archimedean copula models by Wang (2003). Chen (2012) further extended the copula models to implement semi-parametric regression analysis on the transformation Cox model. Several recent works have applied copula-based methods for clustered semi-competing risks data (Emura et al. 2017a, b; Peng et al. 2018).

Nowadays, copulas have been extensively applied for analysis of survival data subject to dependent censoring or competing risks. For a methodological point of view, copulas often offer a more transparent strategy for building a model of dependent censoring and estimating parameters in the model. As an instance, one may compare Clayton's elegant but rather esoteric idea of the conditional likelihood estimation (Clayton 1978) with the more transparent idea of the two-stage likelihood estimation (Shih and Louis 1995). In addition, the likelihood method of Chen (2012) would be more transparent than the moment-type estimating equations of Fine et al. (2001) that were derived under Clayton's model. Indeed, the likelihood method of Chen (2012) is adaptive to more complex copula models, such as the joint frailty-copula model (Emura et al. 2017a, b).

In summary, copulas have provided flexible bivariate survival models to perform survival analysis under dependent censoring. Here, copulas stipulate the dependence structure between event times, while they impose no restriction on the marginal survival models. For these copula-based methods, one can choose any copula that he/she likes, which provides considerable flexibility and adaptability to different types of data. In addition, one can utilize mathematical and computational tools of copulas that have been well-developed in the literature (e.g., Nelsen 2006; Weiß 2011; Joe 2014; Schepsmeier and Stöber 2014; Durante and Sempi 2015).

Remark: There are many articles that we could not mention in this historical review. Our review focuses on likelihood-based inference methods that are of the major interest in this book.

References

Braekers R, Veraverbeke N (2005) A copula-graphic estimator for the conditional survival function under dependent censoring. Can J Stat 33:429–447

Burzykowski T, Molenberghs G, Buyse M (eds) (2005) The evaluation of surrogate endpoints. Springer, New York

Burzykowski T, Molenberghs G, Buyse M, Geys H, Renard D (2001) Validation of surrogate end points in multiple randomized clinical trials with failure time end points. Appl Stat 50(4):405–422

Chen YH (2010) Semiparametric marginal regression analysis for dependent competing risks under an assumed copula. J R Stat Soc Ser B Stat Methodol 72:235–251

Chen YH (2012) Maximum likelihood analysis of semicompeting risks data with semiparametric regression models. Lifetime Data Anal 18:36–57

Clayton DG (1978) A model for association in bivariate life tables and its application in epidemiological studies of familial tendency in chronic disease incidence. Biometrika 65 (1):141–151

Collett D (2015) Modelling survival data in medical research, 3rd edn. CRC Press, London

Cox DR (1972) Regression models and life-tables (with discussion). J R Stat Soc Ser B Stat Methodol 34:187–220

de Uña-Álvarez J, Veraverbeke N (2013) Generalized copula-graphic estimator. TEST 22(2):343–360

de Uña-Álvarez J, Veraverbeke N (2017) Copula-graphic estimation with left-truncated and right-censored data. Statistics 51(2):387–403

Durante F, Sempi C (2015) Principles of copula theory. CRC Press, London

Emura T, Chen YH (2016) Gene selection for survival data under dependent censoring, a copula-based approach. Stat Methods Med Res 25(6):2840–2857

Emura T, Lin CW, Wang W (2010) A goodness-of-fit test for Archimedean copula models in the presence of right censoring. Comput Stat Data Anal 54:3033–3043

Emura T, Nakatochi M, Murotani K, Rondeau V (2017a) A joint frailty-copula model between tumour progression and death for meta-analysis. Stat Methods Med Res 26(6):2649–2666

Emura T, Nakatochi M, Matsui S, Michimae H, Rondeau V (2017b) Personalized dynamic prediction of death according to tumour progression and high-dimensional genetic factors: meta-analysis with a joint model. Stat Methods Med Res. https://doi.org/10.1177/0962280216688032

Emura T, Michimae H (2017) A copula-based inference to piecewise exponential models under dependent censoring, with application to time to metamorphosis of salamander larvae. Environ Ecol Stat 24(1):151–173

Escarela G, Carrière JF (2003) Fitting competing risks with an assumed copula. Stat Methods Med Res 12(4):333–349

Fine JP, Jiang H, Chappell R (2001) On semi-competing risks data. Biometrika 88:907–920

Genest C, MacKay J (1986) The joy of copulas: bivariate distributions with uniform marginals. Am Stat 40(4):280–283

Hsu L, Prentice RL (1996) On assessing the strength of dependency between failure time variates. Biometrika 83:491–506

Joe H (2014) Dependence modeling with copulas. CRC Press, London

Kalbfleisch JD, Prentice RL (2002) The statistical analysis of failure time data, 2nd edn. Wiley, New York

Moradian H, Denis Larocque D, Bellavance F (2017) Survival forests for data with dependent censoring. Stat Methods Med Res. https://doi.org/10.1177/0962280217727314

Nelsen RB (2006) An introduction to copulas, 2nd edn. Springer, New York

Oakes D (1982) A model for association in bivariate survival data. J R Stat Soc Ser B Stat Methodol 414–422

Oakes D (1989) Bivariate survival models induced by frailties. J Am Stat Assoc 84:487–493

Oba K, Paoletti X, Alberts S et al (2013) Disease-free survival as a surrogate for overall survival in adjuvant trials of gastric cancer: a meta-analysis. J Natl Cancer Inst 105(21):1600–1607

Peng M, Xiang L, Wang S (2018) Semiparametric regression analysis of clustered survival data with semi-competing risks. Comput Stat Data Anal 124:53–70

Rivest LP, Wells MT (2001) A martingale approach to the copula-graphic estimator for the survival function under dependent censoring. J Multivar Anal 79:138–155

Schepsmeier U, Stöber J (2014) Derivatives and Fisher information of bivariate copulas. Stat Pap 55(2):525–542

Shih JH, Louis TA (1995). Inferences on the association parameter in copula models for bivariate survival data. Biometrics: 1384–99

Shih JH (1998) A goodness-of-fit test for association in a bivariate survival model. Biometrika 85 (1):189–200

Siannis F, Copas J, Lu G (2005) Sensitivity analysis for informative censoring in parametric survival models. Biostatistics 6(1):77–91

Sklar A (1959) Fonctions de répartition à n dimensions et leurs marges. Publications de l'Institut de Statistique de L'Université de Paris. 8:229–231

Staplin ND (2012) Informative censoring in transplantation statistics. Doctoral thesis, University of Southampton, School of Mathematics

Staplin ND, Kimber AC, Collett D, Roderick PJ (2015) Dependent censoring in piecewise exponential survival models. Statist Methods Med Res 24(3):325–341

Sugimoto T, Hamasaki T, Evans SR (2017) Sizing clinical trials when comparing bivariate time-to-event outcomes. Stat Med 36(9):1363–1382

Tsiatis A (1975) A nonidentifiability aspect of the problem of competing risks. Proc Natl Acad Sci 72(1):20–22

Wang W (2003) Estimating the association parameter for copula models under dependent censoring. J R Stat Soc Series B Stat Methodol 65(1):257–273

Weiß G (2011) Copula parameter estimation by maximum-likelihood and minimum-distance estimators: a simulation study. Comput Stat 26:31–54

Zheng M, Klein JP (1995) Estimates of marginal survival for dependent competing risks based on an assumed copula. Biometrika 82(1):127–138

Chapter 2
Introduction to Survival Analysis

Abstract This chapter provides a concise introduction to survival analysis. We review the essential tools in survival analysis, such as the survival function, Kaplan–Meier estimator, hazard function, log-rank test, Cox regression, and likelihood-based inference.

Keywords Censoring · Cox regression · Independent censoring
Kaplan–Meier estimator · Log-rank test · Overall survival
Time-to-tumor progression

2.1 Survival Time

In survival analysis, the term *survival time* refers to the time elapsed from an origin to the occurrence of an event. In many medical studies, the origin is the time at study entry which can be the start of a medical treatment, the initiation of a randomized experiment, or the operation date of surgery. In epidemiological and demographic studies, the origin is often the date of birth. The event may be the occurrence of death.

In medical research, the term *overall survival* refers to survival time measured from entry until death of a patient. For instance, to measure the effect of chemotherapy or radiotherapy in locally advanced head and neck cancer, researchers may use overall survival as the primary endpoint (Michiels et al. 2009). In this study, the origin is the start of randomization.

2.2 Kaplan–Meier Estimator and Survival Function

We shall introduce the random censorship model where we consider two *random variables*

- T: survival time
- U: censoring time

Due to censoring, either one of T or U is observed. One can observe T if death comes faster than censoring ($T \leq U$). On the other hand, one cannot exactly observe T if censoring comes faster than death ($U < T$). Even if the exact value of T is unknown for the censored case, T is known to be greater than U. What we observe are the first occurring time ($\min\{T, U\}$) and the censoring status ($\{T \leq U\}$ or $\{U < T\}$). The random censorship model typically assumes that T and U are independent, namely $\Pr(T \in A, U \in B) = \Pr(T \in A)\Pr(U \in B)$ for sets A and B.

Survival data consist of (t_i, δ_i), $i = 1, \ldots, n$, where

- t_i: survival time or censoring time whichever comes first,
- δ_i: censoring indicator ($\delta_i = 1$ if t_i is survival time, or $\delta_i = 0$ if t_i is censoring time).

Under the random censorship model, one can write $t_i = \min\{T, U\}$ and $\delta_i = \mathbf{I}(T \leq U)$, where $\mathbf{I}(\cdot)$ is the indicator function. We shall assume that all the observed times to death are distinct ($t_i \neq t_j$ whenever $i \neq j$ and $\delta_i = \delta_j = 1$), so that there is no *ties* in the death times. With the survival data, one can estimate the survival function $S(t) \equiv \Pr(T > t)$ by the following estimator:

Definition 1 *The Kaplan–Meier estimator* (Kaplan and Meier 1958) is defined as

$$\hat{S}(t) = \prod_{t_i \leq t, \delta_i = 1} \left(1 - \frac{1}{n_i}\right), \quad 0 \leq t \leq \max_i(t_i)$$

where $n_i = \sum_{\ell=1}^{n} \mathbf{I}(t_\ell \geq t_i)$ is the *number at-risk* at time t_i; $\hat{S}(t) = 1$ if no death occurs up to time t; $\hat{S}(t)$ is undefined for $t > \max_i(t_i)$.

The derivation of the Kaplan–Meier estimator: Consider a survival function that is a decreasing step function with jumps only at points where a death occurs at observed times of death. Then, one can write (Exercise 1 in Sect. 2.9) the survival function in the form

$$S(t) = \Pr(T > t) = \prod_{t_i \leq t, \delta_i = 1} \left(1 - \frac{\Pr(T = t_i)}{\Pr(T \geq t_i)}\right).$$

Second, suppose that T and U are independent. Then, one can write

$$S(t) = \prod_{t_i \leq t, \delta_i = 1} \left(1 - \frac{\Pr(T = t_i, U \geq t_i)}{\Pr(T \geq t_i, U \geq t_i)}\right)$$

$$= \prod_{t_i \leq t, \delta_i = 1} \left(1 - \frac{\Pr(\min\{T, U\} = t_i, T \leq U)}{\Pr(\min\{T, U\} \geq t_i)}\right).$$

Finally, we replace the probability ratio of the last expression by its estimate to obtain

$$\hat{S}(t) = \prod_{t_i \le t,\, \delta_i = 1} \left(1 - \frac{\sum_{\ell=1}^{n} \mathbf{I}(t_\ell = t_i,\, \delta_\ell = 1)/n}{\sum_{\ell=1}^{n} \mathbf{I}(t_\ell \ge t_i)/n} \right) = \prod_{t_i \le t,\, \delta_i = 1} \left(1 - \frac{1}{n_i} \right).$$

It is now clear that the Kaplan–Meier estimator relies on the independence assumption between T and U. ∎

The Kaplan–Meier survival curve is defined as the plot of $\hat{S}(t)$ against t, starting with $t = 0$ and ending with $t_{\max} = \max_i(t_i)$. The curve is a step function that jumps only at points where a death occurs. On the curve, censoring times are often indicated as the mark "+".

If $t_{\max} = \max_i(t_i)$ corresponds to time-to-death of a patient, then $\hat{S}(t_{\max}) = 0$. If $t_{\max} = \max_i(t_i)$ corresponds to censoring time of a patient, then $\hat{S}(t_{\max}) > 0$. It is misleading to plot $\hat{S}(t)$ only up to the largest death time $\max_{i;\, \delta_i = 1}(t_i)$, especially when many patients are alive beyond $\max_{i;\, \delta_i = 1}(t_i)$.

Survival data often include *covariates*, such as gender, tumor size, and cancer stage. With covariates, survival data consist of $(t_i, \delta_i, \mathbf{x}_i)$, $i = 1, \ldots, n$, where

- $\mathbf{x}_i = (x_{i1}, \ldots, x_{ip})'$: p-dimensional covariates

In traditional survival analysis, the data is analyzed under the following assumption:

Independent censoring assumption: Survival time and censoring time are independent given covariates. That is, T and U are conditionally independent given $\mathbf{x}$.

For a patient i, one can define the *survival function* denoted as $S(t|\mathbf{x}_i) \equiv \Pr(T > t \mid \mathbf{x}_i)$ for $t \ge 0$. The survival function is the probability that the patient is alive at time t. The survival function $S(t|\mathbf{x}_i)$ is, in fact, the *patient-level survival function* as it is conditionally on the patient characteristics $\mathbf{x}_i$. The survival function at $\mathbf{x}_i = \mathbf{0}$ is called the *baseline survival function* and denoted as $S_0(t) = S(t|\mathbf{x}_i = \mathbf{0})$.

A *parametric model* is given by a survival function that is specified by a finite number of parameters. For instance, we consider an exponential survival function

$S(t|x_i) = \exp(-\lambda t e^{\beta x_i})$, $t \geq 0$, where $\lambda > 0$ and $-\infty < \beta < \infty$ are parameters. Let x_i denote the gender with $x_i = 1$ for male and $x_i = 0$ for female. One can show that $S(t|x_i) = S_0(t)^{\exp(\beta x_i)}$ for $t \geq 0$, where $S_0(t) = S(t|x_i = 0) = \exp(-\lambda t)$ is the baseline survival function. With this model, survival difference between male and female is captured by β. The case $\beta > 0$ corresponds to poor survival prognosis for male relative to female; the case $\beta < 0$ corresponds to good survival prognosis for male relative to female. The case $\beta = 0$ corresponds to equal survival prognosis between male and female.

A *semi-parametric model* is given by a survival function that is *partially* specified by a finite number of parameters. For instance, we consider a survival function $S(t|x_i) = S_0(t)^{\exp(\beta x_i)}$, where the form of the baseline survival function $S_0(t)$ is unspecified. In terms of β, one can compare survival between males and females without assuming a specific model on the baseline survival function.

2.3   Hazard Function

Hereafter, we suppose that $S(t|\mathbf{x}_i)$ is a continuous survival function. The instantaneous death probability between t and $t + dt$ is $\Pr(t \leq T < t + dt \mid \mathbf{x}_i) = S(t \mid \mathbf{x}_i) - S(t + dt \mid \mathbf{x}_i)$, where dt is an infinitely small number. Since this probability is equal to zero, one can consider the *rate* by dividing by dt such that

$$f(t \mid \mathbf{x}_i) = \frac{S(t \mid \mathbf{x}_i) - S(t + dt \mid \mathbf{x}_i)}{dt} = \lim_{\Delta t \to 0} \frac{S(t \mid \mathbf{x}_i) - S(t + \Delta t \mid \mathbf{x}_i)}{\Delta t}$$

$$= -\frac{dS(t \mid \mathbf{x}_i)}{dt}.$$

This is the *density function*.

The *hazard rate* describes the instantaneous death rate between t and $t + dt$ given that the patient is at-risk at t:

Definition 2 *The hazard function (or hazard rate function) is defined as*

$$h(t|\mathbf{x}_i) \equiv \frac{\Pr(t \leq T < t + dt \mid T \geq t, \ \mathbf{x}_i)}{dt} = \frac{-\frac{d}{dt} S(t \mid \mathbf{x}_i)}{S(t \mid \mathbf{x}_i)}.$$

The hazard function at $\mathbf{x}_i = \mathbf{0}$ is called the *baseline hazard function* and denoted as $h_0(t) = h(t|\mathbf{x}_i = \mathbf{0})$. The *cumulative hazard function* is defined as $H(t|\mathbf{x}_i) = \int_0^t h(u|\mathbf{x}_i)du$. The survival function is derived from the hazard function through $S(t|\mathbf{x}_i) = \exp\{-H(t|\mathbf{x}_i)\}$.

The hazard rate is also known as the *force of mortality* in actuarial science and demography. For example, let $t =$ "60 years old", $dt =$ "1 year", and $x_i = 1$ for male or $x_i = 0$ for female. Then, the force of mortality $h(60|x_i = 1)$ is equal to the probability of death within the next one year for a 60-year-old man. The Japanese life tables show $h(60|x_i = 1) = 0.0064$ (0.64%). The value of $h(t|x_i = 1)$ monotonically increases as t grows, which represents the effect of natural aging. Eventually, it reaches $h(100|x_i = 1) = 0.3995$ (39.95%). This implies that 40% of Japanese males who have just celebrated their 100th birthday will die before their next birthday. Life tables for almost any country are available in the internet (e.g., Google "Taiwan life table").

Unfortunately, the hazard function for cancer patients in medical studies rarely shows any simple pattern (e.g., monotonically increasing or decreasing). In many clinical trials, the time t is measured from the start of treatment, and hence, the ages are regarded as covariates. In this case, the hazard of patients may be influenced by the treatment effect, the follow-up processes, and cancer progression, so the effect of natural aging may diminish. In epidemiological studies, focusing on age-specific incidence of a particular disease, the time t is measured from birth as in the example from Japanese life tables. However, the shape of the hazard function of disease incidence may be difficult to specify.

This implies that many simple models, such as the exponential, Weibull, and lognormal models, may not fit survival data from cancer patients. This is why semi-parametric models are more useful and widely applied in medical research. One may still accept the assumptions that the hazard function is continuous, does not abruptly change over time, and smooth (continuously differentiable). Hazard models with cubic splines (Chap. 4) meet these assumptions without restricting too much the shape of the hazard function.

The semi-parametric model $S(t|x_i) = S_0(t)^{\exp(\beta x_i)}$ can alternatively be specified in terms of the hazard function

$$h(t|x_i) = h_0(t) \exp(\beta x_i) \tag{2.1}$$

where the form of $h_0(t)$ is unspecified. One can show $h_0(t) = -d\{ \log S_0(t) \}/dt$ and $S_0(t) = \exp\{ -H_0(t) \}$, where $H_0(t) = \int_0^t h_0(u)du$.

Let x_i be a dichotomous covariate, such as gender with $x_i = 1$ for male and $x_i = 0$ for female. Under the model (2.1), the *relative risk* (RR) is defined as

$$RR = \exp(\beta) = \frac{h(t|x_i = 1)}{h(t|x_i = 0)}.$$

For instance, the value $RR = 2$ implies that death rate for $x_i = 1$ is twice the death rate for $x_i = 0$.

Let x_i be a continuous covariate, such as a gene expression. If the scale of x_i is standardized (to be mean $= 0$ and SD $= 1$), then $RR = \exp(\beta)$ is interpreted with respect to one SD increase. If one is interested in the effect of $x_i = 2$ relative to $x_i = -2$, then $RR = \exp(4\beta)$.

2.4 Log-Rank Test for Two-Sample Comparison

The log-rank test is a method to test the quality of the hazard rates between two groups. Specifically, we consider the null hypothesis

$$H_0 : h(t|x_i = 0) = h(t|x_i = 1), \qquad t \geq 0,$$

where $x_i = 1$ for male and $x_i = 0$ for female, for instance. This null hypothesis is the same as the equality $S(t|x_i = 0) = S(t|x_i = 1)$ due to the relationship between the hazard function and survival function. We wish to test H_0 without making any model assumption, but with the assumption that there are no ties in death times. The treatment of ties shall be briefly discussed in Sect. 2.8.

Let $n_{i1} = \sum_{\ell=1}^{n} I\{ t_\ell \geq t_i,\ x_\ell = 1 \}$ be the number of males and $n_{i0} = \sum_{\ell=1}^{n} I\{ t_\ell \geq t_i,\ x_\ell = 0 \}$ be the number of females at-risk at time t_i. Hence, $n_{i0} + n_{i1}$ is the total number at-risk at time t_i. Each death at time t_i corresponds to either the death of male ($x_i = 1$) or the death of female ($x_i = 0$). If there is no effect of gender on survival, male and female have the same death rate. Hence, the conditional expectation of x_i given $(\delta_i = 1, n_{i0}, n_{i1})$ is

$$
\begin{aligned}
E[x_i|\delta_i = 1,\ n_{i0},\ n_{i1}] &= \Pr(x_i = 1|\delta_i = 1,\ n_{i0},\ n_{i1}) \\
&= \frac{\Pr(x_i = 1,\ \delta_i = 1|\ n_{i0},\ n_{i1})}{\Pr(x_i = 1,\ \delta_i = 1|\ n_{i0},\ n_{i1}) + \Pr(x_i = 0,\ \delta_i = 1|\ n_{i0},\ n_{i1})} \\
&= \frac{n_{i1}h(t_i|x_i = 1)}{n_{i1}h(t_i|x_i = 1) + n_{i0}h(t_i|x_i = 0)} \\
&= \frac{n_{i1}}{n_{i0} + n_{i1}}.
\end{aligned}
$$

The last equation holds under the null hypothesis H_0. The difference between x_i and its expectation leads to the *log-rank statistic*

$$S = \sum_{i=1}^{n} \delta_i \left(x_i - \frac{n_{i1}}{n_{i0} + n_{i1}} \right).$$

Hence, $S > 0$ is associated with higher death rate in male than that in female. Under H_0, the mean of S is zero. If we assume that x_i's are independent,

$$Var(S) = \sum_{i=1}^{n} \delta_i \frac{n_{i1} n_{i0}}{(n_{i0} + n_{i1})^2}.$$

The log-rank test for no gender effect is based on the Z-statistic $z = S/\sqrt{Var(S)}$ or the chi-square statistic z^2. The P-value is computed as $Pr(|Z| > |z|)$, where $Z \sim N(0, 1)$.

Example 1 Consider a sample of five females and five males ($n = 10$) with $t_i = (1650, 30, 720, 450, 510, 1110, 210, 1380, 1800, 540)$, $\delta_i = (0, 1, 0, 1, 1, 0, 1, 1, 0, 1)$, and $x_i = (0, 0, 0, 0, 0, 1, 1, 1, 1, 1)$. To calculate the log-rank statistic, it is convenient to summarize the data into Table 2.1.

The log-rank statistic has the "(observed)-(expected)" form, namely

$$S = \sum_{i=1}^{n} \delta_i x_i - \sum_{i=1}^{n} \delta_i \frac{n_{i1}}{n_{i0} + n_{i1}} = 3 - \left(\frac{5}{10} + \frac{5}{9} + \frac{4}{8} + \frac{4}{7} + \frac{4}{6} + \frac{2}{3} \right) = 3 - 3.46$$
$$= -0.46.$$

The negative value of S implies that the observed mortality of male is lower than its expected value under H_0. The variance is computed from Table 2.1 as

$$Var(S) = \sum_{i=1}^{n} \delta_i \frac{n_{i1} n_{i0}}{(n_{i0} + n_{i1})^2} = \frac{5 \times 5}{10^2} + \frac{5 \times 4}{9^2} + \frac{4 \times 4}{8^2} + \frac{4 \times 3}{7^2} + \frac{4 \times 2}{6^2} + \frac{2 \times 1}{3^2}$$
$$= 1.436.$$

Hence, the test statistic is $z = S/\sqrt{Var(S)} = -0.46/\sqrt{1.436} = -0.384$, and the P-value is $Pr(|Z| > 0.384) = 0.70$. We see no significant evidence for gender effect on survival. ∎

The log-rank test is a non-parametric test that does not employ any distributional assumption. The log-rank test simply examines the excess mortality. Software packages for survival analysis display both "observed" and "expected" numbers of deaths in their outputs, in addition to the Z-value and P-value. The log-rank test can also handle *left-truncation* (Klein and Moeschberger 2003). The log-rank test has

Table 2.1 Tabulation of the $n = 10$ samples

Death times: t_i with $\delta_i = 1$	Observed: x_i	Expected: $n_{i1}/(n_{i0} + n_{i1})$
30	0	5/10
210	1	5/9
450	0	4/8
510	0	4/7
540	1	4/6
1380	1	2/3

variants, such as multi-group tests, log-rank trend tests, and stratified log-rank tests (Collett 2003; Klein and Moeschberger 2003).

2.5 Cox Regression

Since the hazard function is the basis of the risk comparison between two groups, it is then natural to incorporate the effect of covariates into the hazard function.

Definition 3 *The Cox proportional hazards model (Cox 1972) is defined as*

$$h(t|\mathbf{x}_i) = h_0(t) \exp(\boldsymbol{\beta}'\mathbf{x}_i),$$

where $\boldsymbol{\beta} = (\beta_1, \ldots, \beta_p)'$ *are unknown coefficients and* $h_0(\cdot)$ *is an unknown baseline hazard function.*

The Cox model states that the hazard function $h(t|\mathbf{x}_i)$ is proportional to $h_0(t)$ with the relative risk $\exp(\boldsymbol{\beta}'\mathbf{x}_i)$. This implies that all patients share the same time-trend function $h_0(t)$. The most striking feature of the Cox model is that the form of $h_0(\cdot)$ is unspecified. Hence, the Cox model is a semi-parametric model, offering greater flexibility over parametric models that specify the form of $h(t|\mathbf{x}_i)$.

One can estimate $\boldsymbol{\beta}$ without estimating $h_0(\cdot)$. Based on data $(t_i, \delta_i, \mathbf{x}_i)$, $i = 1, \ldots, n$, let $R_i = \{ \ell : t_\ell \geq t_i \}$ be the *risk set* that contains patients at-risk at time t_i. The *partial likelihood estimator* $\hat{\boldsymbol{\beta}} = (\hat{\beta}_1, \ldots, \hat{\beta}_p)'$ is defined by maximizing the *partial likelihood function* (Cox 1972)

$$L(\boldsymbol{\beta}) = \prod_{i=1}^{n} \left(\frac{\exp(\boldsymbol{\beta}'\mathbf{x}_i)}{\sum_{\ell \in R_i} \exp(\boldsymbol{\beta}'\mathbf{x}_\ell)} \right)^{\delta_i}.$$

The log-partial likelihood is

$$\ell(\boldsymbol{\beta}) = \log L(\boldsymbol{\beta}) = \sum_{i=1}^{n} \delta_i \left[\boldsymbol{\beta}'\mathbf{x}_i - \log \left\{ \sum_{\ell \in R_i} \exp(\boldsymbol{\beta}'\mathbf{x}_\ell) \right\} \right]. \tag{2.2}$$

The derivatives of $\ell(\boldsymbol{\beta})$ give the *score function*,

$$\mathbf{S}(\boldsymbol{\beta}) = \frac{\partial \ell(\boldsymbol{\beta})}{\partial \boldsymbol{\beta}} = \sum_{i=1}^{n} \delta_i \left[\mathbf{x}_i - \frac{\sum_{\ell \in R_i} \mathbf{x}_\ell \exp(\boldsymbol{\beta}'\mathbf{x}_\ell)}{\sum_{\ell \in R_i} \exp(\boldsymbol{\beta}'\mathbf{x}_\ell)} \right].$$

The second-order derivatives of $\ell(\boldsymbol{\beta})$ constitute the *Hessian matrix*,

$$H(\boldsymbol{\beta}) = \frac{\partial^2 \ell(\boldsymbol{\beta})}{\partial \boldsymbol{\beta} \partial \boldsymbol{\beta}'} = -\sum_{i=1}^{n} \delta_i \left[\frac{\sum_{\ell \in R_i} \mathbf{x}_\ell \mathbf{x}'_\ell \exp(\boldsymbol{\beta}' \mathbf{x}_\ell)}{\sum_{\ell \in R_i} \exp(\boldsymbol{\beta}' \mathbf{x}_\ell)} - \frac{\sum_{\ell \in R_i} \mathbf{x}_\ell \exp(\boldsymbol{\beta}' \mathbf{x}_\ell)}{\sum_{\ell \in R_i} \exp(\boldsymbol{\beta}' \mathbf{x}_\ell)} \left\{ \frac{\sum_{\ell \in R_i} \mathbf{x}_\ell \exp(\boldsymbol{\beta}' \mathbf{x}_\ell)}{\sum_{\ell \in R_i} \exp(\boldsymbol{\beta}' \mathbf{x}_\ell)} \right\}' \right].$$

Since $H(\boldsymbol{\beta})$ is a negative definite matrix (see Exercise 3 in Sect. 2.9), the log-likelihood $\ell(\boldsymbol{\beta})$ is concave. This implies that $\ell(\boldsymbol{\beta})$ has a unique maxima $\hat{\boldsymbol{\beta}}$ that solves $\mathbf{S}(\boldsymbol{\beta}) = \mathbf{0}$.

Interval estimation for $\boldsymbol{\beta}$ is implemented by applying the asymptotic theory (Fleming and Harrington 1991). The *information matrix* is defined as $i(\hat{\boldsymbol{\beta}}) = -H(\hat{\boldsymbol{\beta}})$. The standard error (SE) of $\hat{\beta}_j$ is $SE(\hat{\beta}_j) = \sqrt{\{ i^{-1}(\hat{\boldsymbol{\beta}}) \}_{jj}}$ that uses the j-th diagonal element of the inverse information matrix. The 95% confidence interval (CI) is $\hat{\beta}_j \pm 1.96 \times SE(\hat{\beta}_j)$.

To gain more insight into Cox regression, we consider a simple case where x_i denote the gender defined as $x_i = 1$ for male and $x_i = 0$ for female. In this setting, the Cox model is written as $h(t|x_i) = h_0(t) \exp(\beta x_i)$, where the factor $\exp(\beta)$ represents the RR of male relative to female.

We shall demonstrate how the factor $\exp(\beta)$ is estimated by maximizing the log-partial likelihood in Eq. (2.2). We solve the score equation $S(\beta) = 0$ where

$$S(\beta) = \sum_{i=1}^{n} \delta_i \left[x_i - \frac{\sum_{\ell \in R_i} x_\ell \exp(\beta x_\ell)}{\sum_{\ell \in R_i} \exp(\beta x_\ell)} \right] = \sum_{i=1}^{n} \delta_i \frac{x_i n_{i0} - (1 - x_i) n_{i1} \exp(\beta)}{n_{i0} + n_{i1} \exp(\beta)}.$$

Hence, the estimate of $\exp(\beta)$ needs to satisfy the equation

$$\exp(\beta) = \frac{\sum\limits_{i:x_i=1} \delta_i \frac{n_{i0}}{n_{i0} + n_{i1} \exp(\beta)}}{\sum\limits_{i:x_i=0} \delta_i \frac{n_{i1}}{n_{i0} + n_{i1} \exp(\beta)}}. \tag{2.3}$$

This is the ratio of the expected number of deaths in male divided by the expected number of deaths in female, which agrees with the interpretation of $\exp(\beta)$.

Equation (2.3) can be solved by the *fixed-point iteration algorithm*. First, applying the initial value $\exp(\beta) = 1$ to the right-hand side of Eq. (2.3), we have

$$\exp(\beta) = \frac{\sum\limits_{i:x_i=1} \delta_i \frac{n_{i0}}{n_{i0} + n_{i1}}}{\sum\limits_{i:x_i=0} \delta_i \frac{n_{i1}}{n_{i0} + n_{i1}}}.$$

We apply this value of $\exp(\beta)$ to the right-hand side of Eq. (2.3) to give an updated value of $\exp(\beta)$. This process is repeated until the updated value does not change from the previous step. While the fixed-point iteration gives us an insight about how $\exp(\beta)$ is estimated from data, it requires a large number of iterations until convergence.

A computationally faster algorithm is the *Newton–Raphson algorithm*, which utilizes the score function $S(\beta) = d\ell(\beta)/d\beta$ and the Hessian $H(\beta) = d^2\ell(\beta)/d\beta^2$. The algorithm starts with the initial value $\beta^{(0)} = 0$, and then follows the sequence

$$\beta^{(k+1)} = \beta^{(k)} - H^{-1}(\beta^{(k)})S(\beta^{(k)}), \quad k = 0, 1, \ldots$$

The algorithm converges if $|\beta^{(k+1)} - \beta^{(k)}| \approx 0$. Then, the estimate is $\hat{\beta} = \beta^{(k)}$ and its standard error is $SE(\hat{\beta}) = \sqrt{-H^{-1}(\hat{\beta})}$. The score function is

$$S(\beta) = \sum_{i=1}^{n} \delta_i \left[x_i - \frac{\sum_{\ell \in R_i} x_\ell \exp(\beta x_\ell)}{\sum_{\ell \in R_i} \exp(\beta x_\ell)} \right] = \sum_{i=1}^{n} \delta_i \left[x_i - \frac{n_{i1} \exp(\beta)}{n_{i0} + n_{i1} \exp(\beta)} \right],$$

and the Hessian is

$$H(\beta) = -\sum_{i=1}^{n} \delta_i \left[\frac{\sum_{\ell \in R_i} x_\ell^2 \exp(\beta x_\ell)}{\sum_{\ell \in R_i} \exp(\beta x_\ell)} - \left\{ \frac{\sum_{\ell \in R_i} x_\ell \exp(\beta x_\ell)}{\sum_{\ell \in R_i} \exp(\beta x_\ell)} \right\}^2 \right]$$

$$= -\sum_{i=1}^{n} \delta_i \frac{n_{i0} n_{i1} \exp(\beta)}{\{ n_{i0} + n_{i1} \exp(\beta) \}^2}.$$

We use Example 1 to compare the convergence between the fixed-point iteration and Newton–Raphson algorithms. Table 2.2 shows that the Newton–Raphson converges faster than the fixed-point iteration. The two algorithms reach the same value $\hat{\beta} = -0.3156$.

The Wald test for the null hypothesis $H_0 : \beta = 0$ is based on the Z-value $z = \hat{\beta}/SE(\hat{\beta})$. The P-value is computed as $\Pr(|Z| > |z|)$, where $Z \sim N(0, 1)$.

The score test for the null hypothesis $H_0 : \beta = 0$ uses the score statistic, and its variance,

$$S(0) = \sum_{i=1}^{n} \delta_i \left(x_i - \frac{n_{i1}}{n_{i0} + n_{i1}} \right), \quad Var\{ S(0) \} = -H(0) = \sum_{i=1}^{n} \delta_i \frac{n_{i1} n_{i0}}{(n_{i0} + n_{i1})^2}.$$

Table 2.2 Iteration algorithms to compute $\hat{\beta}$ using the data of Example 1

Iteration number k	Fixed-point iteration $\beta^{(k)}$	Newton–Raphson $\beta^{(k)}$
0	0	0
1	−0.3093212	−0.3204982
2	−0.3154621	−0.3155884
3	−0.3155858	–

Note The convergence criterion is $|\beta^{(k+1)} - \beta^{(k)}| \leq 10^{-5}$

The score test based on $z = S(0)/\sqrt{Var\{\,S(0)\,\}}$ is exactly the same as the log-rank test. This coincidence does not imply that the log-rank test relies on the Cox model assumption (Sect. 2.8).

The Newton–Raphson algorithm can also be applied to the multi-dimensional case ($p \geq 2$) (see Sect. 2.7). The fixed-point iteration algorithm, however, may not be easily applied to the multi-dimensional case (see Exercise 4 in Sect. 2.9).

2.6   R Survival Package

We shall briefly introduce the R package *survival* to analyze real data. After installing the package, we enter survival time t_i, censoring indicator δ_i, and covariate x_i for $n = 10$ patients. Then, we run the codes:

```
library(survival)
t.event=c(1650, 30, 720, 450, 510, 1110,  210, 1380, 1800, 540)
event=c(0, 1, 0, 1, 1, 0, 1, 1, 0, 1)
x=c(0,0,0,0,0,1,1,1,1,1)  ## female=0, male=1
survdiff(Surv(t.event, event) ~ x)  ## log-rank test
summary( coxph(Surv(t.event,event)~x) ) ## Cox regression
fit=survfit(Surv(t.event, event)~1) ## Kaplan-Meier estimator
plot(fit,mark.time=TRUE) ## Kaplan-Meier survival curve
```

The outputs are shown below and Fig. 2.1.

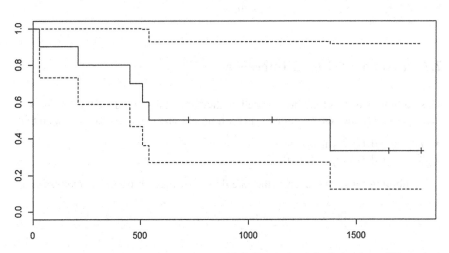

Fig. 2.1 Kaplan–Meier survival curve and the 95% CI calculated from the data of Example 1 ($n = 10$). Censoring times are indicated as the mark"+"

```
> survdiff(Surv(t.event, event) ~ x)  ## log-rank test
Call:
survdiff(formula = Surv(t.event, event) ~ x)
        N  Observed  Expected  (O-E)^2/E   (O-E)^2/V
x=0     5         3      2.54     0.0834       0.148
x=1     5         3      3.46     0.0612       0.148
 Chisq= 0.1  on 1 degrees of freedom, p= 0.701
> summary( coxph(Surv(t.event,event)~x) ) ## Cox regression
Call:
coxph(formula = Surv(t.event, event) ~ x)
  n= 10,  number of events= 6
      coef   exp(coef)  se(coef)      z   Pr(>|z|)
x -0.3156     0.7294    0.8249   -0.383    0.702


   exp(coef)  exp(-coef)  lower .95  upper .95
x    0.7294       1.371     0.1448      3.673


Concordance= 0.581  (se = 0.123 )
Rsquare= 0.014   (max possible= 0.898 )
Likelihood ratio test= 0.15  on 1 df,  p=0.7026
Wald test          = 0.15  on 1 df,  p=0.702
Score (logrank) test = 0.15  on 1 df,  p=0.7009
```

The results on the log-rank test show $S = 3 - 3.46 = -0.46$ with the chi-square statistics $z^2 = 0.148$ and the P-value = 0.701 (see the row of "x = 1"). The results on Cox regression show $\hat{\beta} = -0.316$, $RR = \exp(\hat{\beta}) = 0.729$, $SE(\hat{\beta}) = 0.825$, and $z = \hat{\beta}/SE(\hat{\beta}) = -0.38$. The P-value of the Wald test is 0.702. Hence, the log-rank test and the Wald test show similar results. In addition, the log-rank test and the score test yield the identical result.

Since the difference between the two groups is not significant, we combine the two groups and then draw the Kaplan–Meier survival curve. Figure 2.1 display the Kaplan–Meier survival curve and the 95% CI.

2.7 Likelihood-Based Inference

This section considers likelihood-based methods for analyzing the data (t_i, δ_i, $\mathbf{x}_i$), $i = 1, \ldots, n$. Recall that we defined survival time T and censoring time U such that:

- $T = t_i$ and $U > t_i$ if $\delta_i = 1$,
- $T > t_i$ and $U = t_i$ if $\delta_i = 0$.

Combining these two events, the likelihood for the i-th patient is expressed as

$$L_i = \Pr(T = t_i, \ U > t_i | \mathbf{x}_i)^{\delta_i} \Pr(T > t_i, \ U = t_i | \mathbf{x}_i)^{1-\delta_i}.$$

Under the independent censoring assumption,

$$L_i = [\,\Pr(\,T = t_i|\mathbf{x}_i\,)\Pr(\,U > t_i|\mathbf{x}_i\,)\,]^{\delta_i}[\,\Pr(\,T > t_i|\mathbf{x}_i\,)\Pr(\,U = t_i|\mathbf{x}_i\,)\,]^{1-\delta_i}$$
$$= [\,f_T(t_i|\mathbf{x}_i)S_U(t_i|\mathbf{x}_i)\,]^{\delta_i}[\,S_T(t_i|\mathbf{x}_i)f_U(t_i|\mathbf{x}_i)\,]^{1-\delta_i}$$
$$= [\,f_T(t_i|\mathbf{x}_i)^{\delta_i}S_T(t_i|\mathbf{x}_i)^{1-\delta_i}\,][\,f_U(t_i|\mathbf{x}_i)^{1-\delta_i}S_U(t_i|\mathbf{x}_i)^{\delta_i}\,]$$

where $S_T(t|\mathbf{x}_i) = \Pr(\,T > t \mid \mathbf{x}_i\,)$, $f_T(t|\mathbf{x}_i) = -dS_T(t|\mathbf{x}_i)/dt$, $S_U(t|\mathbf{x}_i) = \Pr(\,U > t \mid \mathbf{x}_i\,)$, and $f_U(t|\mathbf{x}_i) = -dS_U(t|\mathbf{x}_i)/dt$. In addition to the independent censoring assumption, we further impose the following assumption:

Non-informative censoring assumption: *The censoring distribution does not involve any parameters related to the distribution of the survival times. That is, $S_U(t|\mathbf{x}_i)$ does not contain parameters related to $S_T(t|\mathbf{x}_i)$.*

Under the non-informative censoring assumption, the term $f_U(t_i|\mathbf{x}_i)^{1-\delta_i}S_U(t_i|\mathbf{x}_i)^{\delta_i}$ is unrelated to the likelihood for the survival times and can simply be ignored. Therefore, the likelihood function is re-defined as

$$L = \prod_{i=1}^{n} f_T(t_i|\mathbf{x}_i)^{\delta_i}S_T(t_i|\mathbf{x}_i)^{1-\delta_i} = \prod_{i=1}^{n} h_T(t_i|\mathbf{x}_i)^{\delta_i}\exp[\,-H_T(t_i|\mathbf{x}_i)\,],$$

where $h_T(t|\mathbf{x}_i) = f_T(t|\mathbf{x}_i)/S_T(t|\mathbf{x}_i)$ and $H_T(t|\mathbf{x}_i) = \int_0^t h_T(u|\mathbf{x}_i)du$. The log-likelihood is

$$\ell = \log L = \sum_{i=1}^{n}[\,\delta_i\log h_T(t_i|\mathbf{x}_i) - H_T(t_i|\mathbf{x}_i)\,]. \tag{2.4}$$

Usually, censoring is non-informative if it is independent. Only an artificial or unusual example yields informative but independent censoring (p. 150 of Andersen et al. 1993; p. 196 of Kalbfleisch and Prentice 2002). It is well-known that independent censoring is more crucial assumption than non-informative censoring that does not lead to bias in estimation. Throughout the book, we focus on dependent censoring rather than informative censoring.

If censoring is dependent, the likelihood for the i-th patient is

$$L_i = \Pr(\,T = t_i,\ U > t_i|\mathbf{x}_i\,)^{\delta_i}\Pr(\,T > t_i,\ U = t_i|\mathbf{x}_i\,)^{1-\delta_i}$$
$$= \left\{-\frac{\partial}{\partial x}\Pr(\,T > x,\ U > t_i|\mathbf{x}_i\,)\Big|_{x=t_i}\right\}^{\delta_i}\left\{-\frac{\partial}{\partial y}\Pr(\,T > t_i,\ U > y|\mathbf{x}_i\,)\Big|_{y=t_i}\right\}^{1-\delta_i}.$$

Therefore, the log-likelihood is defined as

$$\ell = \sum_{i=1}^{n} [\delta_i \log h_T^{\#}(t_i|\mathbf{x}_i) + (1 - \delta_i) \log h_U^{\#}(t_i|\mathbf{x}_i) - \Phi(t_i, \ t_i|\mathbf{x}_i)],$$

where

$$h_T^{\#}(t_i|\mathbf{x}_i) = -\frac{\partial}{\partial x} \log \Pr(\ T > x, \ U > t_i|\mathbf{x}_i \ )\Big|_{x=t_i},$$

$$h_U^{\#}(t_i|\mathbf{x}_i) = -\frac{\partial}{\partial y} \log \Pr(\ T > t_i, \ U > y|\mathbf{x}_i \ )\Big|_{y=t_i},$$

are the *cause-specific hazard* functions, and

$$\Phi(t_i, \ t_i|\mathbf{x}_i) = -\log \Pr(\ T > t_i, \ U > t_i|\mathbf{x}_i \ ) = -\log \Pr(\ \min\{\ T, \ U \ \} > t_i|\mathbf{x}_i \ )$$

is the cumulative hazard function for $\min\{\ T, \ U \ \}$.

Suppose that the log-likelihood is parameterized by φ. Then, the maximum likelihood estimator (MLE) is defined by maximizing the log-likelihood, $\hat{\varphi} = \arg\max_{\varphi} \ell(\ \varphi\ )$. To find the MLE numerically, one can use the *score function* $S(\ \varphi\ ) = \partial\ell(\ \varphi\ )/\partial\varphi$ and the Hessian matrix $H(\ \varphi\ ) = \partial^2\ell(\ \varphi\ )/\partial\varphi\partial\varphi'$. The MLE $\hat{\varphi}$ is obtained from the Newton–Raphson algorithm

$$\varphi^{(k+1)} = \varphi^{(k)} - H^{-1}(\ \varphi^{(k)}\ )S(\ \varphi^{(k)}\ ), \qquad k = 0, 1, \ldots$$

Interval estimates for φ follow from the asymptotic theory of MLEs. The *information matrix* is defined as $i(\ \hat{\varphi}\ ) = -H(\ \hat{\varphi}\ )$. The SE for $\hat{\varphi}_j$ (the j-th component of $\hat{\varphi}$) is $SE(\hat{\varphi}_j) = \sqrt{\{\ i^{-1}(\hat{\varphi})\ \}_{jj}}$ that uses the j-th diagonal element of the inverse information matrix. The 95% CI is $\hat{\varphi}_j \pm 1.96 \times SE(\hat{\varphi}_j)$.

For instance, the Cox model takes the form $\varphi = (\theta, \beta)$ and $h(t|\mathbf{x}_i) = h_0(t; \theta) \exp(\beta'\mathbf{x}_i)$, where $\theta = (\theta_1, \ldots, \theta_m)$ is a vector of parameters related to the baseline hazard function. We assume that the baseline cumulative hazard function $H_0(t; \theta)$ is an increasing step function with jumps $dH_0(t; \theta) = e^{\theta_j}$ at $t = t_i$ with $\delta_i = 1$. Hence, the number of parameters in θ is equal to the number of deaths $m = \sum_{i=1}^{n} \delta_i$. The MLE $\hat{\varphi} = (\hat{\theta}, \hat{\beta})$ is obtained from the Newton–Raphson algorithm. It has been shown that $\hat{\beta}$ is equivalent to the partial likelihood estimator and $\hat{\theta}$ is the Breslow estimator $h_0(t_j; \hat{\theta}) = e^{\hat{\theta}_j} = \left(\sum_{t_\ell \geq t_j} e^{\hat{\beta}'\mathbf{x}_\ell}\right)^{-1}$ (van der Vaart 1998; van Houwelingen and Putter 2011).

2.8 Technical Notes

Readers can skip this section as it does not influence the understanding of the latter chapters of the book.

The log-rank test possesses an easy-to-understand optimality criterion. The log-rank test is *asymptotically efficient (most powerful)* to detect the constant hazard ratio $h(t|x_i = 1)/h(t|x_i = 0) = \psi$ for some $\psi \neq 1$. Any reasonable test, such as the t-test, has optimality criteria to detect some specific form. The details on the asymptotic efficiency are referred to Andersen et al. (1993) and Fleming and Harrington (1991).

If the form of $h(t|x_i = 1)/h(t|x_i = 0)$ is non-constant, then the log-rank test may be sub-optimal. For example, Gehan's generalized Wilcoxon test statistic (Gehan 1965) defined as

$$S = \sum_{i=1}^{n} \delta_i (n_{i0} + n_{i1}) \left(x_i - \frac{n_{i1}}{n_{i0} + n_{i1}} \right)$$

can be more powerful than the log-rank statistic if the ratio $h(t|x_i = 1)/h(t|x_i = 0)$ strongly deviates from 1 in the early stage of follow-up. The generalized Wilcoxon test statistic is a special case of the *weighted log-rank statistics* (Fleming and Harrington 1991; Klein and Moeschberger 2003). If there is a concern about the non-constant hazard ratio, the weighted log-rank statistics may be employed.

A gross misunderstanding is that the log-rank test is a test tailored to detect the effect in a proportional hazards assumption. As mentioned earlier, the log-rank statistic is a non-parametric test to detect excess mortality without any model assumption.

We have derived the Kaplan–Meier estimator and the log-rank test under the assumption that all times to death are distinct (no ties). To handle ties, it is useful to introduce counting process formulations (Andersen et al. 1993; Fleming and Harrington 1991). For $k = 0, 1$, let $\bar{Y}_k(t) = \sum_{\ell=1}^{n} \mathbf{I}\{ t_\ell \geq t, \ x_\ell = k \}$ be the number at-risk at time t, and let $\bar{N}_k(t) = \sum_{\ell=1}^{n} \mathbf{I}\{ t_\ell \leq t, \ \delta_\ell = 1, \ x_\ell = k \}$ be the number of deaths up to time t. Then, at time t, the number of deaths in male is $d\bar{N}_1(t) = \sum_{\ell=1}^{n} \mathbf{I}\{ t_\ell = t, \ \delta_\ell = 1, \ x_\ell = 1 \}$, and the total number of deaths is $d\bar{N}(t) = \sum_{\ell=1}^{n} \mathbf{I}\{ t_\ell = t, \ \delta_\ell = 1 \}$.

The Kaplan–Meier estimator for the group k is defined as

$$\hat{S}_k(t) = \prod_{u \leq t} \{ 1 - d\hat{H}_k(u) \}, \quad k = 0, 1,$$

where $d\hat{H}_k(t) = d\bar{N}_k(t)/\bar{Y}_k(t)$ is called the *Nelson–Aalen estimator*.

The conditional distribution of $d\bar{N}_1(t)$ given ($d\bar{N}(t)$, $\bar{Y}_0(t)$, $\bar{Y}_1(t)$) is a hyper-geometric distribution with mean

$$E\{ \, d\bar{N}_1(t) | d\bar{N}(t), \ \bar{Y}_0(t), \ \bar{Y}_1(t) \, \} = \frac{d\bar{N}(t)\bar{Y}_1(t)}{\bar{Y}_0(t) + \bar{Y}_1(t)}.$$

Consequently, the aggregated differences between the observed and expected deaths is

$$S = \int_0^\infty \left[d\bar{N}_1(t) - \frac{d\bar{N}(t)\bar{Y}_1(t)}{\bar{Y}_0(t) + \bar{Y}_1(t)} \right] = \int_0^\infty d\bar{N}_1(t) - \int_0^\infty \frac{d\bar{N}(t)\bar{Y}_1(t)}{\bar{Y}_0(t) + \bar{Y}_1(t)}.$$

The univariate partial likelihood estimator as derived in Eq. (2.3) has a counting process form

$$\exp(\hat{\beta}) = \frac{\int_0^\infty W(\hat{\beta}; t) d\hat{H}_1(t)}{\int_0^\infty W(\hat{\beta}; t) d\hat{H}_0(t)}, \quad W(t; \beta) = \frac{\bar{Y}_0(t)\bar{Y}_1(t)}{\bar{Y}_0(t) + \bar{Y}_1(t) \exp(\beta)}.$$

This means that the estimator is the ratio of the expected number of deaths in male divided by the expected number of deaths in female. This way of interpreting the univariate estimator is suggested in Emura and Chen (2016) to argue the robustness of the estimator against the model misspecification. Under the independent censoring assumption, $\hat{\beta}$ is a consistent estimator for β^* that is the solution to

$$\exp(\beta) = \frac{\int_0^\infty w(\beta; t) h(t|x = 1) dt}{\int_0^\infty w(\beta; t) h(t|x = 0) dt}, \quad W(t; \beta) = \frac{\pi_0(t)\pi_1(t)}{\pi_0(t) + \pi_1(t) \exp(\beta)},$$

where $\pi_k(t) = \lim_{n \to \infty} \bar{Y}_k(t)/n$ and the integral is on the range of t with $\pi_0(t)\pi_1(t) > 0$. If the proportional hazards model $h(t|x_i = 1) = \exp(\beta_0)h(t|x_i = 0)$ holds for some β_0, then $\beta^* = \beta_0$. Even if the proportional hazards model does not hold, β^* is still meaningful since $\exp(\beta^*)$ is interpreted as the RR. However, the interpretation of the partial likelihood estimator may not be robust against the violation of the independent censoring assumption (Chap. 3).

2.9 Exercises

1. *Deriving the Kaplan–Meier estimator:* Consider a survival function $S(t) = \Pr(T > t)$ that is a decreasing step function with steps at observed times of death. Assume that all the observed times to death are distinct ($t_i \neq t_j$ whenever $i \neq j$ and $\delta_i = \delta_j = 1$).

(1) Show $\Pr(T > t_i) = \Pr(T > t_i | T > t_{i-1}) \Pr(T > t_{i-1})$ if $t_i > t_{i-1}$.

(2) Show $\Pr(\,T > t_j\,) = \prod_{i=1}^{j} \Pr(\,T > t_i | T > t_{i-1}\,)$ if $t_j > t_{j-1} > \cdots > t_1 > t_0 \equiv 0$
and $S(\,0\,) = 1$.

(3) Show $\Pr(\,T > t_i | T > t_{i-1}\,) = 1 - \Pr(\,T = t_i | T \geq t_i\,)$ if there is no death in the interval $(t_{i-1},\, t_i)$.

(4) Show $S(\,t_j\,) = \prod_{i=1}^{j} \left(1 - \frac{\Pr(T = t_i)}{\Pr(T \geq t_i)}\right)$.

2. *Weibull regression:* Let $\log(T_i) = \alpha_0 + \alpha' \mathbf{x}_i + \sigma \varepsilon_i$, where $\Pr(\varepsilon_i > x) = \exp(-e^x)$ for $-\infty < x < \infty$.

(1) Derive the survival function $S(t | \mathbf{x}_i)$ and the hazard function $h(t | \mathbf{x}_i)$.
(2) Show that the model can be expressed as $h(t | \mathbf{x}_i) = h_0(t) \exp(\boldsymbol{\beta}' \mathbf{x}_i)$.
(3) Show $\Pr(T > t + w | T > t,\, \mathbf{x}_i) < \Pr(T > w | \mathbf{x}_i)$ for $0 < \sigma < 1$ and $w > 0$. What does this inequality imply?

3. Consider a discrete random vector $\mathbf{X}_i = (X_{i1}, \ldots, X_{ip})$ whose distribution is given by

$$\Pr(\mathbf{X}_i = \mathbf{x}_k) = \frac{\exp(\boldsymbol{\beta}' \mathbf{x}_k)}{\sum_{\ell \in R_i} \exp(\boldsymbol{\beta}' \mathbf{x}_\ell)}, \quad k \in R_i = \{\ell : t_\ell \geq t_i\}, \quad i = 1, \ldots, n.$$

This represents the risk of the k-th patient relative to the total risk for those who are at-risk of death at time t_i. By assuming the independence of the sequence $\mathbf{X}_i$, $i = 1, \ldots, n$, one can obtain the partial likelihood function $L(\boldsymbol{\beta}) = \prod_{i=1}^{n} \Pr(\mathbf{X}_i = \mathbf{x}_i)^{\delta_i}$.

(1) Express the score function $\mathbf{S}(\boldsymbol{\beta})$ using $E(\mathbf{X}_i)$.
(2) Express the Hessian matrix $H(\boldsymbol{\beta})$ using $Var(\mathbf{X}_i)$.
(3) Discuss the conditions to make $H(\boldsymbol{\beta})$ negative definite.

4. Suppose that data $(\,t_i,\, \delta_i,\, x_i\,)$, $i = 1, \ldots, n$, follow the model $S(t | x_i) = \exp(\,-\lambda t e^{\beta x_i}\,)$, where $\lambda > 0$ and $-\infty < \beta < \infty$. Let $m = \sum_{i=1}^{n} \delta_i$ be the number of deaths.

(1) Write down the log-likelihood function $\ell(\lambda,\, \beta) = \log L(\lambda,\, \beta)$.
(2) Derive the score functions $\partial \ell(\lambda,\, \beta)/\partial \lambda$ and $\partial \ell(\lambda,\, \beta)/\partial \beta$.
(3) Derive the fixed-point iteration algorithm and apply it to the data of Example 1.
(4) Derive the Hessian matrix of $\ell(\lambda,\, \beta)$.
(5) Derive the Newton–Raphson algorithm and apply it to the data of Example 1.
(6) Derive the Newton–Raphson algorithm under the transformed parameter $\tilde{\lambda} = \log(\lambda)$ and apply it to the data of Example 1.
(7) Compare the numbers of iterations in all the three algorithms.

5. Use the lung cancer data available in the *compound.Cox* R package (Emura et al. 2018) to:

(1) Perform univariate Cox regression treating the *ZNF264* gene or the *NF1* gene as a covariate. Are these genes univariately associated with survival?
(2) Perform multivariate Cox regression treating both the *ZNF264* and *NF1* genes as covariates. Are these genes associated with survival?
(3) Discuss the influence of multicollinearity between *ZNF264* and *NF1*.

References

Andersen PK, Borgan O, Gill RD, Keiding N (1993) Statistical models based on counting processes. Springer, New York

Collett D (2003) Modelling survival data in medical research, 2nd edn. CRC Press, London

Cox DR (1972) Regression models and life-tables (with discussion). J R Stat Soc Ser B Stat Methodol 34:187–220

Emura T, Chen YH (2016) Gene selection for survival data under dependent censoring, a copula-based approach. Stat Methods Med Res 25(6):2840–2857

Emura T, Chen HY, Matsui S, Chen YH (2018) Compound.Cox: univariate feature selection and compound covariate for predicting survival. CRAN

Fleming TR, Harrington DP (1991) Counting processes and survival analysis. Wiley

Gehan EA (1965) A generalized Wilcoxon test for comparing arbitrarily singly-censored samples. Biometrika 52:203–224

Kalbfleisch JD, Prentice RL (2002) The statistical analysis of failure time data, 2nd edn. Wiley, New York

Kaplan EL, Meier P (1958) Nonparametric estimation from incomplete observations. J Am Stat Assoc 53(282):457–481

Klein JP, Moeschberger ML (2003) Survival analysis techniques for censored and truncated data. Springer, New York

Michiels S, Le Maître A, Buyse M, Burzykowski T, Maillard E, Bogaerts J, Pignon JP (2009) Surrogate endpoints for overall survival in locally advanced head and neck cancer: meta-analyses of individual patient data. Lancet Oncol 10(4):341–350

van der Vaart AW (1998) Asymptotic statistics. Cambridge series in statistics and probabilistic mathematics. Cambridge University Press, Cambridge

van Houwelingen HC, Putter H (2011) Dynamic prediction in clinical survival analysis. CRC Press, New York

Chapter 3
Copula Models for Dependent Censoring

Abstract This chapter provides mathematical infrastructures for copula models, focusing on applications to survival analysis involving dependent censoring. After reviewing the concept of copulas, we introduce measures of dependence, including Kendall's tau and the cross-ratio function. We also introduce the idea of *residual dependence* that explains how dependence between event times arises and how it can be modeled by copulas. Finally, we apply copulas for modeling the effect of dependent censoring and analyze the bias of the Cox regression analysis owing to dependent censoring.

Keywords Archimedean copula · Clayton's copula · Cox regression
Cross-ratio function · Gumbel's copula · Kendall's tau · Residual dependence
Univariate Cox regression

3.1 Introduction

Roughly speaking, a *copula* is a function to link two random variables by specifying their dependence structure. The word *copula* is a Latin word that means *bond*, *link*, or *tie* (Nelsen 2006), where *co* means *together*. A mathematician, Abe Sklar, first used the word *copula* in his study of *probabilistic metric space* (Sklar 1959). In his paper, he gave a mathematical definition of copulas and established the most fundamental theorem about copulas, known as *Sklar's theorem*. The full history of copulas can be found in the book of Nelsen (2006).

This chapter provides a mathematical background for bivariate copula models that have been used in survival analysis. Let T be survival time, U be censoring time, and $\mathbf{x}$ be a vector of covariates. Also, let $S_T(t|\mathbf{x}) = \Pr(T > t|\mathbf{x})$ and $S_U(u|\mathbf{x}) = \Pr(U > u|\mathbf{x})$ be the marginal survival functions given $\mathbf{x}$. We consider a bivariate survival function

$$\Pr(T > t, U > u|\mathbf{x}) = C_\theta\{S_T(t|\mathbf{x}), S_U(u|\mathbf{x})\}, \tag{3.1}$$

© The Author(s) 2018   27
T. Emura and Y.-H. Chen, *Analysis of Survival Data with Dependent Censoring*,
JSS Research Series in Statistics, https://doi.org/10.1007/978-981-10-7164-5_3

where a function C_θ is called copula (Nelsen 2006) and a parameter θ describes the degree of dependence between T and U. With this model, the dependency between T and U is described by C_θ. As we shall detail in Sect. 3.2, the copula function C_θ must satisfy certain mathematical conditions such that Eq. (3.1) becomes a valid survival function.

Kendall's tau (τ) is a well-known measure to assess the dependence between T and U, which is defined by

$$\tau = \Pr\{ (T_2 - T_1)(U_2 - U_1) > 0 | \mathbf{x} \} - \Pr\{ (T_2 - T_1)(U_2 - U_1) < 0 | \mathbf{x}\},$$

where (T_1, U_1) and (T_2, U_2) are drawn from the model (3.1). Remarkably, Kendall's tau is solely expressed as a function of C_θ through

$$\tau_\theta = 4 \int_0^1 \int_0^1 C_\theta(u, v) C_\theta(du, dv) - 1.$$

This expression implies that Kendall's tau does not depend on the marginal survival functions. The copula model (3.1) has a number of other mathematical properties that are useful for modeling dependent censoring.

This chapter is organized as follows. Sections 3.2 and 3.3 describe the definition and fundamental properties of copulas. Section 3.4 explains the concept of residual dependence. Section 3.5 applies copulas to analyze the bias of the Cox regression analysis owing to dependent censoring.

3.2 Bivariate Copula

This section provides a concise introduction to copulas.

A *bivariate copula* is defined as a bivariate distribution function whose marginal distributions are the uniform distribution on $[0, 1]$. Let $C_\theta : [0, 1]^2 \mapsto [0, 1]$ be a bivariate copula indexed by a parameter θ. By the definition, any bivariate copula satisfies the following conditions

(C1) $C_\theta(u, 0) = C_\theta(0, v) = 0$, $C_\theta(u, 1) = u$, and $C_\theta(1, v) = v$ for $0 \le u \le 1$ and $0 \le v \le 1$.

(C2) $C_\theta(u_2, v_2) - C_\theta(u_2, v_1) - C_\theta(u_1, v_2) + C_\theta(u_1, v_1) \ge 0$ for $0 \le u_1 \le u_2 \le 1$ and $0 \le v_1 \le v_2 \le 1$.

Condition (C1) requires the uniformity of the two marginal distributions. Condition (C2) requires that C_θ produces a probability mass on the rectangular region $[u_1, u_2] \times [v_1, v_2]$.

For a copula C_θ, one can consider a pair of random variables (V, W) such that $\Pr(V \leq u, W \leq v) = C_\theta(u, v)$. If one defines a pair of random variables (T, U) by setting $T = S_T^{-1}(V|\mathbf{x})$ and $U = S_U^{-1}(W|\mathbf{x})$, its bivariate survival function satisfies Eq. (3.1).

Now suppose that C_θ has the density function defined as

$$C_\theta^{[1,1]}(u, v) = \frac{\partial^2}{\partial u \partial v} C_\theta(u, v) \quad \text{for} \quad 0 \leq u \leq 1 \quad \text{and} \quad 0 \leq v \leq 1.$$

Then, Condition (C2) is equivalent to the condition of the nonnegative density:

(C2') $\quad C_\theta^{[1,1]}(u, v) \geq 0$ for $0 \leq u \leq 1$ and $0 \leq v \leq 1$.

Condition (C2) implies Condition (C2') since

$$\frac{\partial^2}{\partial u \partial v} C_\theta(u, v) = \lim_{\substack{\Delta u \to 0 \\ \Delta v \to 0}} \frac{C_\theta(u + \Delta u, v + \Delta v) - C_\theta(u + \Delta u, v) - C_\theta(u, v + \Delta v) + C_\theta(u, v)}{\Delta u \Delta v}.$$

Condition (C2') implies Condition (C2) since

$$C_\theta(u, v) = \int_0^u \int_0^v \frac{\partial^2}{\partial s \partial t} C_\theta(s, t) ds dt.$$

The following copulas meet Conditions (C1) and (C2):

The independence copula:

$$C(u, v) = uv,$$

The Clayton copula (Clayton 1978):

$$C_\theta(u, v) = (u^{-\theta} + v^{-\theta} - 1)^{-1/\theta}, \qquad \theta > 0,$$

The Gumbel copula (Gumbel 1960), also known as the Hougaard copula:

$$C_\theta(u, v) = \exp\left[-\{(-\log u)^{\theta+1} + (-\log v)^{\theta+1}\}^{\frac{1}{\theta+1}}\right], \qquad \theta \geq 0,$$

The Frank copula (Frank 1979):

$$C_\theta(u, v) = -\frac{1}{\theta}\log\left\{1 + \frac{(e^{-\theta u} - 1)(e^{-\theta v} - 1)}{e^{-\theta} - 1}\right\}, \quad \theta \neq 0.$$

The Joe copula (Joe 1993):

$$C_\theta(u, v) = 1 - \{(1 - u)^\theta + (1 - v)^\theta - (1 - u)^\theta(1 - v)^\theta\}^{1/\theta}, \quad \theta \geq 1,$$

The Farlie–Gumbel–Morgenstern (FGM) copula (Morgenstern 1956):

$$C(u, v) = uv\{1 + \theta(1 - u)(1 - v)\}, \quad -1 \leq \theta \leq 1.$$

Figure 3.1 gives the scatter plots for (T_i, U_i), $i = 1, \ldots, 500$, under the Clayton copula model with the standard exponential distribution defined as

$$\Pr(T_i > t, U_i > u) = \{(e^{-t})^{-\theta} + (e^{-u})^{-\theta} - 1\}^{-1/\theta}, \quad \text{for} \quad \theta = 2 \text{ and } \theta = 8.$$

These data were generated by setting $T_i = -\log V_i$ and $U_i = -\log W_i$, where (V_i, W_i), $i = 1, \ldots, 500$, were generated from the Clayton copula. The plots exhibit positive dependence between T_i and U_i, where the levels of dependence are different between $\theta = 2$ and $\theta = 8$.

An *Archimedean copula* is defined as

$$C_\theta(u, v) = \phi_\theta^{-1}\{\phi_\theta(u) + \phi_\theta(v)\},$$

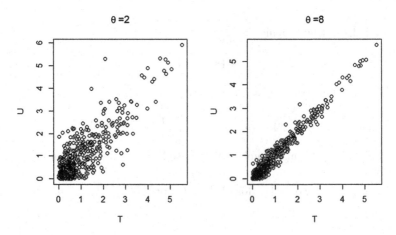

Fig. 3.1 Scatter plots of $n = 500$ pairs generated from the standard exponential distribution under the Clayton copula with $\theta = 2$ ($\tau_\theta = 0.5$) and $\theta = 8$ ($\tau_\theta = 0.8$)

where the function $\phi_\theta : [0, 1] \mapsto [0, \infty]$ is called a *generator* of the copula, which is continuous and strictly decreasing from $\phi_\theta(0) > 0$ to $\phi_\theta(1) = 0$. If $\phi_\theta(0) \equiv \lim_{t \downarrow 0} \phi_\theta(t) = \infty$, the generator function ϕ_θ is called a *strict generator* and has the inverse function $\phi_\theta^{-1} : [0, \infty] \mapsto [0, 1]$ (p. 112 of Nelsen 2006). Under these conditions, C_θ satisfies Condition (C1). To meet Condition (C2), the generator ϕ_θ must be a convex function. Therefore, it suffices to assume $d\phi_\theta(t)/dt < 0$ and $d^2 \phi_\theta(t)/dt^2 > 0$ for any $t \in (0, 1)$, $\phi_\theta(1) = 0$, and $\phi_\theta(0) = \infty$. The proof verifying Conditions (C1) and (C2) under these assumptions is referred to Theorem 4.1.4 of Nelsen (2006).

The Clayton copula has a strict generator $\phi_\theta(t) = (t^{-\theta} - 1)/\theta$ for $\theta > 0$. The limit

$$\lim_{\theta \to 0} \phi_\theta(t) = \lim_{\theta \to 0} \frac{t^{-\theta} - t^{-0}}{\theta} = \frac{d}{d\theta} t^{-\theta}\Big|_{\theta=0} = -\log(t)$$

is also a strict generator corresponding to the independence copula. Thus, $\lim_{\theta \to 0} C_\theta(u, v) = uv$ under the Clayton copula.

The Clayton copula can be extended to the range $-1 \leq \theta < 0$ with some modification. In this case, the generator is non-strict since $\phi_\theta(0) = -1/\theta < \infty$. A mathematical inconvenience is that the domain of ϕ_θ^{-1} is restricted to $[0, -1/\theta]$. This drawback is remedied by extending the domain by defining the *pseudo-inverse* $\phi_\theta^{-1}(t) = \{\max(0, \theta t + 1)\}^{-1/\theta}$ for $t \geq 0$ (Definition 4.1.1 of Nelsen 2006). Consequently, the Clayton copula can be extended as

$$C_\theta(u, v) = \begin{cases} (u^{-\theta} + v^{-\theta} - 1)^{-1/\theta} & \text{if } \theta > 0, \\ uv & \text{if } \theta = 0, \\ \{\max(u^{-\theta} + v^{-\theta} - 1, 0)\}^{-1/\theta} & \text{if } -1 < \theta < 0. \end{cases}$$

The negative-parameter Clayton copula is occasionally useful (e.g., Emura et al. 2011).

Table 3.1 summarizes the generator functions of the Clayton, Gumbel, Frank, and Joe copulas. These four copulas have a strict generator function. The FGM copula does not have a generator function as it is not an Archimedean copula.

3.3 Dependence Measures

Let (V, W) be a pair of random variables such that $\Pr(V \leq u, W \leq v) = C_\theta(u, v)$. *Kendall's tau* is a measure of dependence between V and W, defined as

Table 3.1 Examples of copulas

	Parameter	Generator: $\phi_\theta(t)$	Kendall's tau: τ_θ	$r_\theta(s) = -s\phi_\theta''(s)/\phi_\theta'(s)$
Clayton	$\theta > 0$	$(t^{-\theta} - 1)/\theta$	$\theta/(\theta+2)$	$1 + \theta$
Gumbel	$\theta \geq 0$	$\{-\log(t)\}^{\theta+1}$	$\theta/(\theta+1)$	$1 - \theta/\log(s)$
Frank	$\theta \neq 0$	$-\log\left(\dfrac{e^{-\theta t} - 1}{e^{-\theta} - 1}\right)$	$1 - \frac{4}{\theta}\left(1 - \frac{1}{\theta}\int_0^\theta \frac{t}{e^t-1}dt\right)$	$\dfrac{s\theta}{1 - e^{-\theta s}}$
Joe	$\theta \geq 1$	$-\log\{1 - (1-t)^\theta\}$	$1 - 4\int_0^\infty \frac{t(1-e^{-t})^{2/\theta-2}e^{-2t}}{\theta^2}dt$	$\dfrac{s}{1-s}\left[\dfrac{\theta}{1-(1-s)^\theta} - 1\right]$
FGM	$-1 \leq \theta \leq 1$	None	$2\theta/9$	None

$$\tau_\theta = \Pr\{(V_2 - V_1)(W_2 - W_1) > 0\} - \Pr(\{V_2 - V_1)(W_2 - W_1) < 0\},$$

where (V_1, W_1) and (V_2, W_2) have the same distribution as (V, W). It can be shown that

$$\tau_\theta = 4\int_0^1\int_0^1 C_\theta(u, v)C_\theta(du, dv) - 1 = 4\int_0^1\int_0^1 C_\theta(u, v)C_\theta^{[1,1]}(u, v)dudv - 1.$$

For instance, under the FGM copula, one can calculate the above integral to compute $\tau_\theta = 2\theta/9$ for $-1 \leq \theta \leq 1$. This means that the range of τ_θ under the FGM copula is limited to the interval between $-2/9$ and $2/9$.

An Archimedean copula has a simpler form

$$\tau_\theta = 1 + 4\int_0^1 \frac{\phi_\theta(t)}{\phi_\theta'(t)}dt = 1 - 4\int_0^\infty s\left\{\frac{d}{ds}\phi_\theta^{-1}(s)\right\}^2 ds.$$

Table 3.1 summarizes τ_θ for the Clayton, Gumbel, Frank, and Joe copulas. In these copulas, τ_θ increases with θ and $\tau_\theta \to 1$ as $\theta \to \infty$.

It is convenient to define partial derivatives of a copula:

$$C_\theta^{[1,0]}(u, v) = \frac{\partial}{\partial u}C_\theta(u, v), \quad C_\theta^{[0,1]}(u, v) = \frac{\partial}{\partial v}C_\theta(u, v),$$

$$C_\theta^{[1,1]}(u, v) = \frac{\partial^2}{\partial u \partial v}C_\theta(u, v).$$

The *cross-ratio* function (Oakes 1989) is defined as

$$R_\theta(u, v) = \frac{C_\theta^{[1,1]}(u, v)C_\theta(u, v)}{C_\theta^{[1,0]}(u, v)C_\theta^{[0,1]}(u, v)}.$$

Under the independence copula, $R_\theta(u, v) = 1$ for $0 \leq u \leq 1$ and $0 \leq v \leq 1$. Remarkably, the Clayton copula has the constant cross-ratio $R_\theta(u, v) = 1 + \theta$. The cross-ratio function describes the *local dependence* at a location (u, v):

- $R_\theta(u, v) > 1$: positive local dependence,
- $0 < R_\theta(u, v) < 1$: negative local dependence,
- $R_\theta(u, v) = 1$: local independence.

A simplified formula of the cross-ratio function is available for an Archimedean copula. Using basic derivative rules, it can be shown that

$$R_\theta(u, v) = r_\theta\{C_\theta(u, v)\},$$

where $r_\theta(s) = -s\phi''_\theta(s)/\phi'_\theta(s)$. Table 3.1 shows the formulas for $r_\theta(\cdot)$ under selected copulas. Hence, the cross-ratio function depends on (u, v) only through a one-dimensional quantity $s = C_\theta(u, v)$. Oakes (1989) obtained an inverse formula to obtain $\phi_\theta(\cdot)$ from $r_\theta(\cdot)$.

The cross-ratio function has a practical interpretation as the relative risk (RR). Consider a medical follow-up in which the endpoint is time-to-death T. A patient may drop out at time U due to reasons such as treatment toxicity and tumor progression (informative dropout). We are interested in how the timing of dropout influences the risk of death. For this purpose, we evaluate the influence of dropout using the *conditional hazard functions*:

- $h_T(t|U = u, \mathbf{x}) = \Pr(t \leq T < t + dt | T \geq t, U = u, \mathbf{x})/dt$:

  - the hazard function of death given that a patient has dropped out at time u

- $h_T(t|U > u, \mathbf{x}) = \Pr(t \leq T < t + dt | T \geq t, U > u, \mathbf{x})/dt$:

  - the hazard function of death given that a patient has not yet dropped out at time u

Under a model $\Pr(T > t, U > u|\mathbf{x}) = C_\theta\{S_T(t|\mathbf{x}), S_U(u|\mathbf{x})\}$, the RR is expressed as

$$\frac{h_T(t|U = u, \mathbf{x})}{h_T(t|U > u, \mathbf{x})} = R_\theta\{S_T(t|\mathbf{x}), S_U(u|\mathbf{x})\}.$$

If $R_\theta > 1$, patients who have dropped out at time u possess higher risk of death compared to those who have not yet dropped out at time u. The Clayton copula yields the constant RR for any t and u and hence is regarded as a type of proportional hazard models.

The usefulness of the cross-ratio function is not restricted to the case where U is the time of dropout and T is time-to-death. One may define U as a predictive biomarker for cancer recurrence and T as time-to-recurrence (Day et al. 1997). Emura et al. (2017a, b) considered the case where U is time-to-tumor progression and T is time-to-death under their joint frailty-copula model. If we define U as the delayed entry time (left-truncation time), the cross-ratio function is useful to assess the degree of dependent truncation (Emura et al. 2011). The issues of dependent truncation shall be shortly discussed in the final chapter of this book.

We have seen that the Clayton copula has nice properties for statistical modeling: (1) a simple copula function, (2) simple expression of Kendall's tau, (3) constant cross-ratio function, and (4) interpretability of the parameter θ as the RR. These properties are extremely useful for modeling bivariate survival data and interpreting the results of data analysis.

3.4   Residual Dependence

This section introduces the concept of *residual dependence* between survival time and censoring time. Residual dependence arises when some important covariates influencing both survival time and censoring time are ignored or omitted during the analysis of data. This idea was considered by Clayton (1978) when he introduced his bivariate survival model.

In the Cox model $h(t|\mathbf{x}) = h_0(t) \exp(\boldsymbol{\beta}'\mathbf{x})$, the regression coefficients $\boldsymbol{\beta}$ are estimated by the partial likelihood estimator. The consistency of the estimator critically relies on the *independent censoring assumption* represented as

$$\Pr(T > t, U > u|\mathbf{x}) = S_T(t|\mathbf{x})S_U(u|\mathbf{x}), \tag{3.2}$$

where $S_T(t|\mathbf{x}) = \Pr(T > t|\mathbf{x})$ and $S_U(u|\mathbf{x}) = \Pr(U > u|\mathbf{x})$ are   the   survival functions.

Suppose that a two-dimensional vector of covariates $\mathbf{x} = (x_1, x_2)'$ relates to both T and U. Further suppose that a researcher is interested in the effect of x_1 on survival. If a researcher performs univariate Cox regression by treating x_1 as a single covariate while omitting x_2, the required independent censoring assumption is

$$\Pr(T > t, U > u|x_1) = S_T(t|x_1)S_U(u|x_1),$$

where $S_T(t|x_1) = \Pr(T > t|x_1)$ and $S_U(u|x_1) = \Pr(U > u|x_1)$ are the marginal survival functions given x_1. However, one usually cannot verify the independent censoring assumption given only x_1 even if Eq. (3.2) holds for $\mathbf{x} = (x_1, x_2)'$.

Figure 3.2 explains how the independent censoring assumption fails to hold by omitting x_2. Since x_2 relates to both T and U, the variation in x_2 induces random effects, a popular idea to introduce dependence in bivariate survival models (Oakes 1989). For instance, if x_2 is a gene expression predictive of tumor progression, a higher (lower) value of x_2 is linked to shorter (longer) values of T and U. Consequently, T and U exhibit positive association.

The above discussions lead to a principle that the independent censoring assumption is less likely to hold if many important covariates are omitted or ignored

Fig. 3.2 Mechanism of yielding residual dependence between survival time and censoring time by omitting a covariate

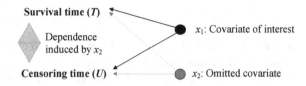

from the Cox model. This mechanism of yielding dependence is termed *residual dependence*. In particular, the independent censoring assumption may not be fulfilled for Cox regression with only one covariate (univariate Cox regression). Residual dependence may arise in a meta-analysis where important covariates are missing in some studies (Emura et al. 2017a, b).

The mechanism of yielding residual dependence in univariate Cox regression is seen by using mathematical expressions as follows. Suppose that T and U are conditionally independent given $\mathbf{x}$, that is, Eq. (3.2) holds. Assume the Cox models $\Pr(T > t|\mathbf{x}) = \exp\{-e^{\boldsymbol{\beta}'\mathbf{x}}\Lambda_T(t)\}$ and $\Pr(U > u|\mathbf{x}) = \exp\{-e^{\boldsymbol{\gamma}'\mathbf{x}}\Lambda_U(u)\}$,   where $\Lambda_T(t)$ and $\Lambda_U(u)$ are cumulative hazard functions. Let $X_j = e^{\boldsymbol{\beta}'_{(-j)}\mathbf{x}_{(-j)}}$ and $Y_j = e^{\boldsymbol{\gamma}'_{(-j)}\mathbf{x}_{(-j)}}$, where $\boldsymbol{\beta}_{(-j)}$ is $\boldsymbol{\beta}$ excluding β_j; similarly $\boldsymbol{\gamma}_{(-j)}$ and $\mathbf{x}_{(-j)}$ are defined. Thus, the bivariate survival function is assumed to be $\Pr(T > t, U > u|\mathbf{x}) = \exp\{-e^{\beta_j x_j}\Lambda_T(t)X_j - e^{\gamma_j x_j}\Lambda_U(u)Y_j\}$. It follows that, for a given x_j (the jth component of $\mathbf{x}$),

$$\Pr(T > t, U > u|x_j) = \varphi_{\boldsymbol{\beta}(-j),\boldsymbol{\gamma}(-j)}[\varphi^{-1}_{\boldsymbol{\beta}(-j)}\{\Pr(T > t\,|x_j)\}, \varphi^{-1}_{\boldsymbol{\gamma}(-j)}\{\Pr(U > u\,|x_j)\}]$$

(3.3)

where $\varphi_{\boldsymbol{\beta}(-j),\boldsymbol{\gamma}(-j)}(u, v) = E\{\exp(-uX_j - vY_j)|x_j\}$, $\varphi_{\boldsymbol{\beta}(-j)}(u) = \varphi_{\boldsymbol{\beta}(-j),\boldsymbol{\gamma}(-j)}(u, 0)$, and $\varphi_{\boldsymbol{\gamma}(-j)}(v) = \varphi_{\boldsymbol{\beta}(-j),\boldsymbol{\gamma}(-j)}(0, v)$ are Laplace transforms. For a special case where $\boldsymbol{\beta} = \boldsymbol{\gamma}$, we obtain an *Archimedean copula* model

$$\Pr(T > t, U > u|x_j) = \varphi_{\boldsymbol{\beta}(-j)}[\varphi^{-1}_{\boldsymbol{\beta}(-j)}\{\Pr(T > t|x_j)\} + \varphi^{-1}_{\boldsymbol{\beta}(-j)}\{\Pr(U > u\,|x_j)\}].$$

(3.4)

The above analysis indicates that the model (3.2) yields dependency between T and U given only x_j. Hence,

$$\Pr(T > t, U > u|x_j) = \Pr(T > t|x_j)\Pr(U > u|x_j), \quad j = 1, \ldots, p$$

(3.5)

does not hold in general, which is a more stringent condition than Eq. (3.2).

In general, T and U may be dependent for any given x_j with an unknown dependence structure. Sklar's theorem (Sklar 1959; Nelsen 2006) guarantees that the bivariate survival function is written as

$$\Pr(T > t, U > u|x_j) = C_j\{\Pr(T > t|x_j), \Pr(U > u|x_j)\}, \quad j = 1, \ldots, p,$$

where C_j is a copula. Equation (3.5) corresponds to $C_j(u, v) = uv$ for $j = 1, \ldots, p$. This is clearly a strong assumption in light of Eq. (3.3) or (3.4). Although the form of C_j is difficult to specify, copulas can relax the stringent condition of $C_j(u, v) = uv$ for $j = 1, \ldots, p$. We shall further consider this copula-based method in Chap. 5.

3.5   Biased Estimation of Cox Regression Due to Dependent Censoring

Following Emura and Chen (2016), we shall apply copulas to study biased estimation of Cox regression when dependent censoring exists. Define notations

- T: survival time,
- U: censoring time,
- x: covariate taking 0 or 1.

The conditional independence between T and U given x is not assumed so that T may be dependently censored by U. The hazard function for T is defined as

$$h(t|x) \equiv \Pr(t \leq T < t + dt|T \geq t, x)/dt.$$

Under the univariate Cox model $h(t|x) = h_0(t) \exp(\beta x)$, one can show

$$\beta = \log \frac{h(t|x = 1)}{h(t|x = 0)}.$$

The parameter β is interpreted as the log of hazard ratio comparing $h(t|x = 1)$ and $h(t|x = 0)$. Recall that the partial likelihood estimate of β is essentially equal to the log of observed hazard ratio (Chap. 2). However, under dependent censoring, the observed hazard rates do not correctly capture $h(t|x = 1)$ and $h(t|x = 0)$, and hence, the estimate of β may be biased.

To quantify the bias, we use the *cause-specific hazard* function

$$h^{\#}(t|x) = \Pr(t \leq T < t + dt, T \leq U|T \geq t, U \geq t, x)/dt$$

which describes the *apparent* hazard for death in the presence of dependent censoring (p. 251, Kalbfleisch and Prentice 2002). With dependent censoring, observed survival data give a biased estimate of $h(t|x)$ while they give an asymptotically unbiased estimate of $h^{\#}(t|x)$ (Fleming and Harrington 1991). The equality $h^{\#}(t|x) = h(t|x)$ holds under either one of the following two conditions.

Condition (A): T and U are independent given x (independent censoring assumption).
Condition (B): Survival time is not censored, that is, $\Pr(U < T|x) = 0$.

Otherwise, $h^{\#}(t|\,x)$ and $h(t|\,x)$ are usually different. The larger discrepancy between $h^{\#}(t|\,x)$ and $h(t|\,x)$ corresponds to the stronger effect of dependent censoring on the bias.

Within the counting process theory, the equality $h^{\#}(t|\,x) = h(t|\,x)$ itself is adopted as the formal definition of *independent censoring* (Fleming and Harrington 1991), a slightly weaker assumption than Condition (A).

We shall examine the effect of dependent censoring under a copula model

$$\Pr(T > t, U > u|x) = C_\theta\{S_T(t|x), S_U(u|x)\},$$

where $S_T(t\,|x) = \Pr(\,T > t\,|x\,)$ and $S_U(u\,|x) = \Pr(\,U > u\,|x\,)$ are the marginal survival functions, and C_θ is a copula with a parameter θ. As indicated in Rivest and Wells (2001), the cause-specific hazard function becomes $h_\theta^{\#}(t|\,x) = \gamma_\theta(t|\,x)h(t|x)$, where

$$\gamma_\theta(t|x) = \frac{C_\theta^{[1,0]}\{S_T(t|x), S_U(t|x)\}S_T(t|x)}{C_\theta\{S_T(t|x), S_U(t|x)\}}.$$

This motivates us to define the apparent effect of the covariate x,

$$\beta^{\#}(\theta, t) \equiv \log\frac{h_\theta^{\#}(t|x = 1)}{h_\theta^{\#}(t|x = 0)} = \underbrace{\log\frac{h(t|x = 1)}{h(t|x = 0)}}_{\text{True effect}} + \underbrace{\log\frac{\gamma_\theta(t|x = 1)}{\gamma_\theta(t|x = 0)}}_{\text{Bias}}.$$

The equation shows that the apparent effect can be partitioned into the true effect and the bias. Note that the copula enters into the bias only.

Under the Cox model $h(t|x) = h_0(t)\exp(\beta x)$, one can formulate the bias of estimating β,

$$\text{Bias}(\theta, t) \equiv \beta^{\#}(\theta, t) - \beta = \log\frac{\gamma_\theta(t|x = 1)}{\gamma_\theta(t|x = 0)}.$$

The bias vanishes if $C_\theta(u, v) = uv$. The bias is usually nonzero except for some special copulas. To visualize the effect of the bias, we suggest fixing the value t at the median survival $S_T(t|0) = 0.5$ and plotting $\text{Bias}(\theta, t)$ against θ.

We conducted numerical analysis under the Clayton copula model

$$\Pr(\,T > t\,,\ U > u | x\,) = \{\,S_T(t\,|x)^{-\theta} + S_U(u\,|x)^{-\theta} - 1\,\}^{-1/\theta}, \qquad \theta > 0, \quad (3.6)$$

where $\;S_T(t|x) = S_T(t|0)^{\exp(\beta x)}, \quad S_U(u|x) = S_U(u|0)^{\exp(\beta x)}, \quad$ and $\quad S_U(t\,|0) = S_T(t\,|0)^{pc/(1-pc)}$ for $0 < pc < 1$. Here, $pc \times 100$ (%) is the censoring percentage such that $pc \approx \Pr(U < T | x)$. Then, one can calculate Bias$(\theta,\ t)$ by using

$$\gamma_\theta(t|x) = \frac{S_T(t|x)^{-\theta}}{S_T(t|x)^{-\theta} + S_U(t|x)^{-\theta} - 1} = \frac{\{S_T(t|0)^{\exp(\beta x)}\}^{-\theta}}{\{S_T(t|0)^{\exp(\beta x)}\}^{-\theta} + \{S_U(t|0)^{\exp(\beta x)}\}^{-\theta} - 1}.$$

Figure 3.3 displays Bias$(\theta,\ t)$ under the Clayton copula model when t is fixed such that $S_T(t\,|0) = 0.5$. If the censoring percentage is high (70%), the bias differs substantially from zero. Furthermore, the bias inflates as θ deviates from zero. For the censoring percentages 30 and 50%, the bias is modest. The bias vanishes if the censoring percentage is zero; that is, Bias$(\theta,\ t) = 0$ for any $\theta > 0$.

It is interesting to point out that Bias$(\theta,\ t)$ under the Gumbel copula behaves very differently from that under the Clayton copula. Under the Gumbel copula,

$$\gamma_\theta(t|x) = \{-\log S_T(t|x)\}^\theta [\{-\log S_T(t|x)\}^{\theta+1} + \{-\log S_U(t|x)\}^{\theta+1}]^{-\frac{\theta}{\theta+1}}$$
$$= e^{\theta \beta x} \{-\log S_T(t|0)\}^\theta [e^{(\theta+1)\beta x} \{-\log S_T(t|0)\}^{\theta+1} + e^{(\theta+1)\beta x} \{-\log S_U(t|0)\}^{\theta+1}]^{-\frac{\theta}{\theta+1}}$$
$$= \{-\log S_T(t|0)\}^\theta [\{-\log S_T(t|0)\}^{\theta+1} + \{-\log S_U(t|0)\}^{\theta+1}]^{-\frac{\theta}{\theta+1}}.$$

Hence, $\gamma_\theta(\,t|1\,) = \gamma_\theta(\,t|0\,)$. This implies that Bias$(\theta,\ t) = 0$ for any θ and t.

We wish to compare Bias$(\theta,\ t)$ with the actual bias $E_\theta[\hat{\beta}] - \beta$, where $\hat{\beta}$ is the partial likelihood estimator. To do so, we conducted Monte Carlo simulations. We generated data of $n = 500$ under the Clayton copula model in Eq. (3.6). The

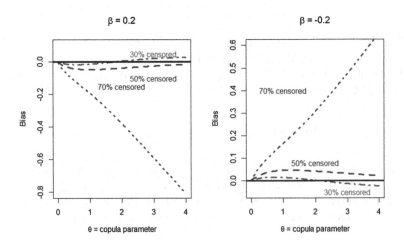

Fig. 3.3 Plot of Bias$(\theta, t) \equiv \beta^\#(\theta, t) - \beta$ under the Clayton copula with parameter θ

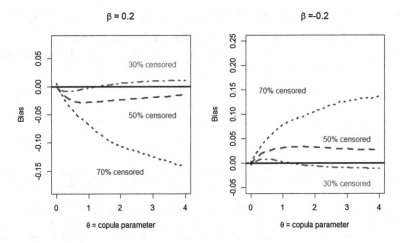

Fig. 3.4 Bias $E_\theta[\hat\beta] - \beta$ under the Clayton copula with parameter θ

marginal survival function is $S_T(t|0) = \exp(-t)$, and the covariate takes $x_i = 0$ or $x_i = 1$ with probability 0.5. All parameter settings followed those for Fig. 3.3. We computed $\hat\beta$ using the data and then calculated $E_\theta[\hat\beta] - \beta$ based on 1000 repetitions. Figure 3.4 shows that $E_\theta[\hat\beta] - \beta$ is very similar to Bias(θ, t). Our additional simulations under the Gumbel copula show that $E_\theta[\hat\beta] - \beta$ is very close to zero which agrees with Bias(θ, t) = 0.

3.6   Exercises

1. Show that Condition (C2') does not hold for $C_\theta(u, v) = (u^{-\theta} + v^{-\theta} - 1)^{-1/\theta}$ with $-1 < \theta < 0$.
2. Verify Conditions (C1) and (C2') for the Clayton, Gumbel, FGM, and Joe copulas.
3. Define a pair of random variables (T, U) by setting $T = S_T^{-1}(V|\mathbf{x})$ and $U = S_U^{-1}(W|\mathbf{x})$, where a pair of random variables (V, W) satisfies $\Pr(V \le u, W \le v) = C_\theta(u, v)$. Show $\Pr(T > t, U > u|\mathbf{x}) = C_\theta\{S_T(t|\mathbf{x}), S_U(u|\mathbf{x})\}$.
4. Show that the copula density for an Archimedean copula is expressed as $C_\theta^{[1,1]}(u, v) = -\phi_\theta''\{C_\theta(u, v)\}\phi_\theta'(u)\phi_\theta'(v)/[\phi_\theta'\{C_\theta(u, v)\}]^3$.
5. Calculate Kendall's tau for the Clayton, Gumbel, FGM, and Joe copulas.
6. Calculate the cross-ratio function R_θ under the Clayton, Gumbel, FGM, and Joe copulas.
7. Verify the equality $h^\#(t|x) = h(t|x)$ under Condition (A) or (B).

8. Let $\quad S_T(t|x) = S_T(t|0)^{\exp(\beta x)}, \quad S_U(u|x) = S_U(u|0)^{\exp(\beta x)}, \quad$ and $\quad S_U(t|0) = S_T(t|0)^{pc/(1-pc)}$. Show $p_C = \Pr(U < T|x)$ under Condition (A).

9. Express $\Pr(U < T|x)$ under the Clayton copula model (3.6). Hint: expression may be in an integral form on $[0, 1]$ (Emura and Pan 2017).

References

Clayton DG (1978) A model for association in bivariate life tables and its application in epidemiological studies of familial tendency in chronic disease incidence. Biometrika 65 (1):141–151

Day R, Bryant J, Lefkopoulou M (1997) Adaptation of bivariate frailty models for prediction, with application to biological markers as prognostic indicators. Biometrika 84(1):45–56

Emura T, Chen YH (2016) Gene selection for survival data under dependent censoring, a copula-based approach. Stat Methods Med Res 25(6):2840–2857

Emura T, Nakatochi M, Murotani K, Rondeau V (2017a) A joint frailty-copula model between tumour progression and death for meta-analysis. Stat Methods Med Res 26(6):2649–2666

Emura T, Nakatochi M, Matsui S, Michimae H, Rondeau V (2017b) Personalized dynamic prediction of death according to tumour progression and high-dimensional genetic factors: meta-analysis with a joint model. Stat Methods Med Res, https://doi.org/10.1177/0962280216688032

Emura T, Pan CH (2017). Parametric likelihood inference and goodness-of-fit for dependently left-truncated data, a copula-based approach. Stat Pap, https://doi.org/10.1007/s00362-017-0947-z

Emura T, Wang W, Hung HN (2011) Semi-parametric inference for copula models for dependently truncated data. Stat Sinica 21:349–367

Fleming TR, Harrington DP (1991) Counting processes and survival analysis. Wiley, New York

Frank MJ (1979) On the simultaneous associativity of $f(x, y)$ and $x + y - f(x, y)$. Aequationes Matbematicae 19:194–226

Gumbel EJ (I960). Distributions de valeurs en plusieurs dimensions. PubL Inst Statist. Parids 9: 171–173

Joe H (1993) Parametric families of multivariate distributions with given margins. J Multivar Anal 46:262–282

Kalbfleisch JD, Prentice RL (2002) The statistical analysis of failure time data, 2nd edn. Wiley, New York

Morgenstern D (1956) Einfache Beispiele zweidimensionaler Verteilungen. Mitteilungsblatt für Mathematishe Statistik. 8:234–235

Nelsen RB (2006) An introduction to copulas, 2nd edn. Springer, New York

Oakes D (1989) Bivariate survival models induced by frailties. J Am Stat Assoc 84:487–493

Rivest LP, Wells MT (2001) A martingale approach to the copula-graphic estimator for the survival function under dependent censoring. J Multivar Anal 79:138–155

Sklar A (1959) Fonctions de répartition à n dimensions et leurs marges. Publications de l'Institut de Statistique de L'Université de Paris. 8:229–231

Chapter 4
Analysis of Survival Data Under an Assumed Copula

Abstract This chapter introduces statistical methods for analyzing survival data subject to dependent censoring. We review the copula-graphic estimator, parametric likelihood methods, and semi-parametric likelihood methods developed under a variety of copula models. All these approaches employ an *assumed copula*, a copula function that is completely specified including its parameter value to avoid the non-identifiability.

Keywords Burr distribution · Competing risk · Copula-graphic estimator
Maximum likelihood estimator · Spline · Weibull distribution

4.1 Introduction

The idea of an *assumed copula* was suggested by Zheng and Klein (1995) in their analysis of survival data subject to dependent censoring. They considered a bivariate distribution function of survival time and censoring time, where the form of the copula function is completely specified, including its parameter value. This strong assumption of the copula is imposed to make the model identifiable. Assuming the independence copula is equivalent to the assumption of independent censoring between survival time and censoring time.

Zheng and Klein (1995) view censoring as a *competing risk* of death and view death as a competing risk of censoring. This is the setting of *bivariate competing risks* where one can observe the first-occurring event time and the type of the observed event (death or censoring whichever comes first). With this view, survival data with dependent censoring are equivalent to bivariate competing risks data. In the context of competing risks, the independence among event times is rarely assumed since many medical and engineering applications yield event times that are positively associated. Hence, statistical methods for analyzing bivariate competing risks data can be applicable for analyzing survival data with dependent censoring.

Under an assumed copula, Zheng and Klein (1995) estimated the marginal survival function by the *copula-graphic* (CG) estimator. The survival function

© The Author(s) 2018
T. Emura and Y.-H. Chen, *Analysis of Survival Data with Dependent Censoring*,
JSS Research Series in Statistics, https://doi.org/10.1007/978-981-10-7164-5_4

estimated by the CG estimator is analogous to the one estimated by the Kaplan–Meier estimator. The CG estimator reduces to the Kaplan–Meier estimator under the independence copula. In real applications, the CG estimator is calculated by assuming one of Archimedean copulas. Rivest and Wells (2001) obtained a simple expression of the CG estimator when the assumed copula belongs to Archimedean copulas. Nowadays, the CG estimator is an indispensable tool for analyzing survival data with dependent censoring (Braekers and Veraverbeke 2005; Staplin 2012; de Uña-Álvarez and Veraverbeke 2013; 2017; Emura and Chen 2016; Emura and Michimae 2017; Moradian et al. 2017). Note, however, that the CG estimator cannot handle covariates. Likelihood-based approaches can naturally deal with covariates under an assumed copula.

Throughout this chapter, we review the copula-graphic estimator, parametric likelihood methods, and semi-parametric likelihood methods developed under an assumed copula.

4.2   The Copula-Graphic (CG) Estimator

Analysis of survival data often begins by drawing the Kaplan–Meier survival curve which graphically summarizes survival experience of patients in the data. However, under dependent censoring, the Kaplan–Meier estimator may give biased information about survival. A survival curve calculated from the CG estimator provides unbiased information about survival if the copula function between death time and censoring time is correctly specified. Below, we shall introduce the CG estimator under an Archimedean copula as derived in Rivest and Wells (2001).

Consider *random variables*, defined as

- T: survival time
- U: censoring time

Consider an Archimedean copula model

$$\Pr(T > t, U > u) = \phi_\theta^{-1}[\phi_\theta\{S_T(t)\} + \phi_\theta\{S_U(u)\}], \tag{4.1}$$

where $\phi_\theta : [0, 1] \mapsto [0, \infty]$ is a generator function, which is continuous and strictly decreasing from $\phi_\theta(0) = \infty$ to $\phi_\theta(1) = 0$ (Chap. 3); $S_T(t) = \Pr(T > t)$ and $S_U(u) = \Pr(U > u)$ are the marginal survival functions.

Let (t_i, δ_i), $i = 1, \ldots, n$, be survival data without covariates, where $t_i = \min\{T_i, U_i\}$, $\delta_i = \mathbf{I}(T_i \le U_i)$, and $\mathbf{I}(\cdot)$ is the indicator function. Assume that all the observed times are distinct ($t_i \ne t_j$ whenever $i \ne j$). Based on the data, one can estimate the survival function by the following estimator:

The CG estimator is defined as

$$\hat{S}_T(t) = \phi_\theta^{-1}\left[\sum_{t_i \le t, \delta_i=1} \phi_\theta\left(\frac{n_i - 1}{n}\right) - \phi_\theta\left(\frac{n_i}{n}\right)\right], \quad 0 \le t \le \max_i(t_i)$$

where $n_i = \sum_{\ell=1}^{n} \mathbf{I}(t_\ell \ge t_i)$ is the *number at risk* at time t_i; $\hat{S}_T(t) = 1$ if no death occurs up to time t; $\hat{S}_T(t)$ is undefined for $t > \max_i(t_i)$.

The derivation of the CG estimator: Assume that $S_T(t)$ is a decreasing step function with jumps at death times. Thus, $\delta_i = 1$ implies $S_T(t_i) \ne S_T(t_i - dt)$ and $S_U(t_i) = S_U(t_i - dt)$. Setting $t = u = t_i$ in Eq. (4.1), we have

$$\phi_\theta\{\Pr(T > t_i, U > t_i)\} = \phi_\theta\{S_T(t_i)\} + \phi_\theta\{S_U(t_i)\}.$$

In the left-side of the preceding equation, we estimate $\Pr(T > t_i, U > t_i)$ by $(n_i - 1)/n$, where $n_i - 1 = \sum_{\ell=1}^{n} \mathbf{I}(t_\ell > t_i)$ is the number of survivors at time t_i. Accordingly,

$$\phi_\theta\left(\frac{n_i - 1}{n}\right) = \phi_\theta\{S_T(t_i)\} + \phi_\theta\{S_U(t_i)\}. \tag{4.2}$$

Meanwhile, we set $t = u = t_i - dt$ in Eq. (4.1) and then estimate $\Pr(T > t_i - dt, U > t_i - dt)$ by n_i/n. Then,

$$\phi_\theta\left(\frac{n_i}{n}\right) = \phi_\theta\{S_T(t_i - dt)\} + \phi_\theta\{S_U(t_i)\}, \quad \delta_i = 1. \tag{4.3}$$

Equations (4.2) and (4.3) result in the system of difference equations

$$\phi_\theta\left(\frac{n_i - 1}{n}\right) - \phi_\theta\left(\frac{n_i}{n}\right) = \phi_\theta\{S_T(t_i)\} - \phi_\theta\{S_T(t_i - dt)\}, \quad \delta_i = 1.$$

We impose the usual constraint that $S_T(t_i - dt) = 1$ when t_i is the smallest death time. Then, the solution to the different equations is

$$\phi_\theta\{S_T(t)\} = \sum_{t_i \le t, \delta_i=1} [\phi_\theta\{S_T(t_i)\} - \phi_\theta\{S_T(t_i - dt)\}]$$

$$= \sum_{t_i \le t, \delta_i=1} \phi_\theta\left(\frac{n_i - 1}{n}\right) - \phi_\theta\left(\frac{n_i}{n}\right),$$

which is equivalent to the CG estimator.   ∎

Under the independence copula, given by $\phi_\theta(t) = -\log(t)$, the CG estimator is equivalent to the Kaplan–Meier estimator. Under the Clayton copula, given by $\phi_\theta(t) = (t^{-\theta} - 1)/\theta$ for $\theta > 0$, the CG estimator is written as

$$\hat{S}_T(t) = \left[1 + \sum_{t_i \le t, \delta_i = 1} \left\{ \left(\frac{n_i - 1}{n}\right)^{-\theta} - \left(\frac{n_i}{n}\right)^{-\theta} \right\} \right]^{-1/\theta}.$$

This CG estimator can be computed by the *compound. Cox* R package (Emura et al. 2018).

The CG estimator provides a graphical summary of survival experience for patients in the same manner as the Kaplan–Meier estimator.

> *The survival curve is defined as the plot of $\hat{S}_T(t)$ against t, starting with t = 0 and ending with $t_{\max} = \max\limits_{i}(t_i)$. The curve is a step function that jumps only at points where a death occurs. On the curve, censoring times are often indicated as the mark "+".*

If $t_{\max} = \max\limits_{i}(t_i)$ corresponds to time-to-death of a patient, then $\hat{S}_T(t_{\max}) = \phi_\theta^{-1}(\infty) = 0$. This is because $\phi_\theta\left(\frac{n_i-1}{n}\right) = \phi_\theta(0) = \infty$ for some i in the definition of the CG estimator. If $t_{\max} = \max\limits_{i}(t_i)$ corresponds to censoring time of a patient, then $\hat{S}(t_{\max}) > 0$.

Additional remarks: The CG estimator can be modified to accommodate a variety of different censoring and truncation mechanisms. de Uña-Álvarez and Veraverbeke (2013) derived the CG estimator when survival time is subject to both dependent censoring and independent censoring. This estimator is convenient if the data provide the causes of censors for all patients. For instance, censoring caused by dropout may be dependent while censoring caused by the study termination is independent (see Chap. 14 of Collett (2015)). de Uña-Álvarez and Veraverbeke (2017) derived the CG estimator when survival time is subject to both dependent censoring and independent truncation. Chaieb et al. (2006) and Emura and Murotani (2015) derived the CG estimator when survival time is subject to independent censoring and *dependent truncation*.

4.3 Model and Likelihood

Throughout this chapter, we consider a bivariate survival function

$$\Pr(T > t, U > u|\mathbf{x}) = C_\theta\{S_T(t|\mathbf{x}), S_U(u|\mathbf{x})\},$$

where C_θ is a copula (Nelsen 2006) with a parameter θ; $S_T(t|\mathbf{x}) = \Pr(T > t|\mathbf{x})$ and $S_U(u|\mathbf{x}) = \Pr(U > u|\mathbf{x})$ are the marginal survival functions. The covariates are defined as $\mathbf{x} = (\mathbf{x}_1, \mathbf{x}_2)$ such that $S_T(t|\mathbf{x}) = S_T(t|\mathbf{x}_1)$ and $S_U(u|\mathbf{x}) = S_U(t|\mathbf{x}_2)$. For instance, if $\mathbf{x}_1 = (\text{Age}, \text{gender})$ and $\mathbf{x}_2 = (\text{gender})$, the model does not consider the effect of age on censoring time.

Survival data consist of $(t_i, \delta_i, \mathbf{x}_i)$, $i = 1, \ldots, n$, where $\mathbf{x}_i = (x_{i1}, \ldots, x_{ip})'$ is a vector of covariates. The likelihood for the ith patient is expressed as

$$L_i = \Pr(T = t_i, U > t_i|\mathbf{x}_i)^{\delta_i} \Pr(T > t_i, U = t_i|\mathbf{x}_i)^{1-\delta_i} = f_T^\#(t_i|\mathbf{x}_i)^{\delta_i} f_U^\#(t_i|\mathbf{x}_i)^{1-\delta_i},$$

where

$$f_T^\#(t_i|\mathbf{x}_i) = -\frac{\partial}{\partial x}\Pr(T > x, U > t_i|\mathbf{x}_i)\Big|_{x=t_i},$$

$$f_U^\#(t_i|\mathbf{x}_i) = -\frac{\partial}{\partial y}\Pr(T > t_i, U > y|\mathbf{x}_i)\Big|_{y=t_i},$$

are called the *sub-density functions*. Therefore, the log-likelihood is defined as

$$\ell = \sum_{i=1}^{n}[\delta_i \log f_T^\#(t_i|\mathbf{x}_i) + (1 - \delta_i) \log f_U^\#(t_i|\mathbf{x}_i)]. \tag{4.4}$$

An equivalent expression is

$$\ell = \sum_{i=1}^{n}[\delta_i \log h_T^\#(t_i|\mathbf{x}_i) + (1 - \delta_i) \log h_U^\#(t_i|\mathbf{x}_i) - \Phi(t_i, t_i|\mathbf{x}_i)], \tag{4.5}$$

where

$$h_T^\#(t_i|\mathbf{x}_i) = \frac{f_T^\#(t_i|\mathbf{x}_i)}{\Pr(T > t_i, U > t_i|\mathbf{x}_i)}, \quad h_U^\#(t_i|\mathbf{x}_i) = \frac{f_U^\#(t_i|\mathbf{x}_i)}{\Pr(T > t_i, U > t_i|\mathbf{x}_i)},$$

are the *cause-specific hazard* functions, and

$$\Phi(t_i, t_i|\mathbf{x}_i) = -\log \Pr(T > t_i, U > t_i|\mathbf{x}_i) = -\log \Pr(\min\{T, U\} > t_i|\mathbf{x}_i)$$

is the cumulative hazard function for $\min\{T, U\}$.

With appropriate models on C_θ, $S_T(\cdot|\mathbf{x})$ and $S_U(\cdot|\mathbf{x})$, one can obtain the maximum likelihood estimator (MLE) with Eqs. (4.4) or (4.5).

4.4   Parametric Models

4.4.1   The Burr Model

Escarela and Carrière (2003) considered a copula model with the Burr distribution defined as

$$S_T(t|\mathbf{x}_{1i}) = \{1 + \gamma_1(\lambda_{1i}t)^{v_1}\}^{-1/\gamma_1}, \quad t \geq 0;$$
$$S_U(u|\mathbf{x}_{2i}) = \{1 + \gamma_2(\lambda_{2i}u)^{v_2}\}^{-1/\gamma_2}, \quad u \geq 0,$$

where $v_j > 0$, $\gamma_j > 0$, and $\lambda_{ji} = \exp(\beta_{j0} + \boldsymbol{\beta}_j'\mathbf{x}_{ji})$ for $j = 1$ and 2. The Burr distribution includes many distributions as special cases; $v_j = 1$ gives the Pareto distribution, $\gamma_j = 1$ gives the log-logistic distribution, and $\gamma_j \to 0$ gives the Weibull distribution. For the copula, Escarela and Carrière (2003) considered the Frank copula.

$$C_\theta(u,v) = -\frac{1}{\theta}\log\left\{1 + \frac{(e^{-\theta u}-1)(e^{-\theta v}-1)}{e^{-\theta}-1}\right\}, \quad \theta \neq 0.$$

Their motivation to use the Frank model is that they wish to consider both positive dependence ($\theta > 0$) and negative dependence ($\theta < 0$) between two variables.

4.4.2   The Weibull Model

Likelihood-based analyses of Escarela and Carrière (2003) focused on the Weibull model

$$S_T(t|\mathbf{x}_{1i}) = \exp\{-(\lambda_{1i}t)^{v_1}\}, \quad t \geq 0; \quad S_U(u|\mathbf{x}_{2i}) = \exp\{-(\lambda_{2i}u)^{v_2}\}, \quad u \geq 0.$$

With the Frank copula model, they maximize the log-likelihood of Eq. (4.4) with respect to $(\beta_{10}, \boldsymbol{\beta}_1, v_1, \beta_{20}, \boldsymbol{\beta}_2, v_2)$ given the value θ. This leads to the profile likelihood

$$\ell^*(\theta) = \max_{(\beta_{10},\boldsymbol{\beta}_1,v_1,\beta_{20},\boldsymbol{\beta}_2,v_2)} \ell(\beta_{10}, \boldsymbol{\beta}_1, v_1, \beta_{20}, \boldsymbol{\beta}_2, v_2|\theta).$$

The MLE of $(\beta_{10}, \boldsymbol{\beta}_1, v_1, \beta_{20}, \boldsymbol{\beta}_2, v_2)$ is obtained at a given value $\hat{\theta} = \arg\max_\theta \ell^*(\theta)$.

The data analysis of Escarela and Carrière (2003) revealed that the estimator $\hat{\theta}$ had a wide confidence interval (CI) if no covariate enters the model. This phenomenon is related to the non-identifiability of the model. The CI of $\hat{\theta}$ was shrunken if many covariates enter the model. Heckman and Honoré (1989) showed that the non-identifiability is resolved by adding covariates into the marginal models. Unfortunately, there are no papers that give the conditions (e.g., how many covariates or how many samples) required to give reasonable precision of $\hat{\theta}$ for estimating the true value θ.

In this context, we suggest regarding the approach of Escarela and Carrière (2003) as a two-step fashion. The first stage *selects* (not *estimates*) θ via the profile likelihood. With the selected value $\hat{\theta}$, the second stage estimates the remaining parameters $(\beta_{10}, \boldsymbol{\beta}_1, \nu_1, \beta_{20}, \boldsymbol{\beta}_2, \nu_2)$ by the MLE. The SEs of $(\beta_{10}, \boldsymbol{\beta}_1, \nu_1, \beta_{20}, \boldsymbol{\beta}_2, \nu_2)$ may not account for the variation of $\hat{\theta}$ following the approaches of an assumed copula.

4.4.3 The Pareto Model

In the absence of covariates, Shih et al. (2018) considered the Pareto marginal models

$$S_T(t) = (1 + \alpha_1 t)^{-\gamma_1}, \quad t \geq 0; \quad S_U(u) = (1 + \alpha_2 u)^{-\gamma_2}, \quad u \geq 0,$$

where $\alpha_j > 0$ and $\gamma_j > 0$ are re-parameterized from the Burr models. The marginal hazard functions are $h_T(t) = \alpha_1 \gamma_1 / (1 + \alpha_1 t)$ and $h_U(u) = \alpha_2 \gamma_2 / (1 + \alpha_2 u)$ and the marginal density functions are $f_T(t) = h_T(t) S_T(t)$ and $f_U(u) = h_U(u) S_U(u)$. Applying the Frank copula to Eq. (4.4), the log-likelihood can be written as

$$\ell(\alpha_1, \alpha_2, \gamma_1, \gamma_2 | \theta) = \sum_{i=1}^{n} \delta_i \{\log f_T(t_i) - \theta S_T(t_i) + \log(e^{-\theta S_T(t_i)} - 1) - \log(e^{-\theta} - 1) + \theta S(t_i)\}$$

$$+ \sum_{i=1}^{n} (1 - \delta_i)\{\log f_U(t_i) - \theta S_U(t_i) + \log(e^{-\theta S_U(t_i)} - 1) - \log(e^{-\theta} - 1) + \theta S(t_i)\},$$

where $S(t) = C_\theta \{S_T(t), S_U(t)\}$. The MLE is obtained by maximizing the preceding equation.

They developed a Newton–Raphson algorithm to obtain the MLE of $(\alpha_1, \alpha_2, \gamma_1, \gamma_2)$ given the value θ. The *Bivariate.Pareto* R package (Shih and Lee 2018) can be used to compute the MLE and the SE for the parameters. Hence, this model uses an assumed copula. Their Newton–Raphson algorithm employs a *randomization* scheme to reduce the sensitivity of the convergence results against the initial values, which is termed the *randomized Newton–Raphson* algorithm (Hu and Emura 2015). When θ is unknown, the profile likelihood estimate was suggested, namely $\hat{\theta} = \arg\max_\theta \ell^*(\theta)$, where $\ell^*(\theta) = \max_{(\alpha_1, \alpha_2, \gamma_1, \gamma_2)} \ell(\alpha_1, \alpha_2, \gamma_1, \gamma_2 | \theta)$.

However, they reported that the profile likelihood occasionally does not have a peak and $\hat{\theta}$ has a large sampling variation. These problems are related to the non-identifiability of competing risks data (Tsiatis 1975).

Due to the difficulty of estimating θ, Shih et al. (2018) considered a restricted model $S_T(t) = S_U(t) = (1 + \alpha t)^{-\gamma}$. The model makes a strong assumption that the two marginal distributions are the same. Under the Frank copula, they developed the randomized Newton–Raphson algorithm to obtain the MLE of (α, γ, θ). While the peak of the likelihood always exists under this restricted model, the variation of estimating θ remains large. Including covariates into the marginal Pareto models may improve the precision of $\hat{\theta}$. Alternatively, a sensitivity analysis may be considered under a few selected values of θ.

4.4.4 The Burr III Model

In the absence of covariates, Shih and Emura (2018) considered the Burr III marginal distributions

$$S_T(t) = 1 - (1 + t^{-\gamma})^{-\alpha}, \quad t > 0; \quad S_U(u) = 1 - (1 + u^{-\gamma})^{-\beta}, \quad u > 0,$$

where (α, β, γ) are positive parameters. They considered the generalized FGM copula with a copula parameter θ. In their model, the copula is imposed on a bivariate distribution function rather than a bivariate survival function. More details about this copula, such as the range of θ and the expressions of Kendall's tau, are referred to Amini et al. (2011), Domma and Giordano (2013) and Shih and Emura (2016, 2018).

Shih and Emura (2018) used the randomized Newton–Raphson algorithm to obtain the MLE of (α, β, γ) given the value of θ. When the value of θ is unknown, they suggested making inference for (α, β, γ), followed by the profile likelihood estimate $\hat{\theta} = \arg\max_\theta \ell^*(\theta)$, where $\ell^*(\theta) = \max_{(\alpha,\beta,\gamma)} \ell(\alpha, \beta, \gamma | \theta)$. They also proposed a goodness-of-fit method to test the validity of the generalized FGM copula and the Burr III marginal models. The estimation and goodness-of-fit algorithms are implemented in the *GFGM.copula* R package (Shih 2018). Their method is developed for bivariate competing risks data, where dependent censoring is a competing risk of death, and death is a competing risk of dependent censoring.

4.4.5 The Piecewise Exponential Model

The piecewise exponential model has been considered to fit survival data with dependent censoring (Staplin et al. 2015; Emura and Michimae 2017). Let $0 = \alpha_0 < a_1 < \cdots < a_m$ be a knot sequence, where m is the number of knots. Assume that the hazard function for T in an interval $(a_{j-1}, a_j]$ is a constant e^{θ_j} for $j = 1, \ldots, m$, such that $\theta = (\theta_1, \ldots, \theta_m)$ are parameters without restriction to their ranges. The survival function is

$$S_T(t; \theta) = \exp\left\{ -e^{\theta_j}(t - a_{j-1}) - \sum_{k=1}^{j-1} e^{\theta_k}(a_k - a_{k-1}) \right\}, \qquad t \in (a_{j-1}, a_j],$$

where $\sum_{k=1}^{0}(\cdot) \equiv 0$. In a similar fashion, define the survival function $S_U(u; \gamma)$ for the censoring time U, where $\gamma = (\gamma_1, \ldots, \gamma_m)$.

Emura and Michimae (2017) considered a copula model

$$\Pr(T > t, U > u) = C_\theta\{S_T(t; \theta), S_U(u; \gamma)\}, \quad \theta = (\theta_1, \ldots, \theta_m), \gamma = (\gamma_1, \ldots, \gamma_m),$$

where $S_T(t; \theta)$ and $S_U(u; \gamma)$ follow the piecewise exponential models. The Clayton copula and the Joe copula were chosen for their numerical studies. They developed inference procedures based on the likelihood in Eq. (4.4) given the value θ. Hence, they applied an assumed copula. They did not use the profile likelihood for selecting θ since it may not work with many parameters in the marginal distributions. Alternatively, they suggested a sensitivity analysis to examine the result under a few different values of θ.

Staplin et al. (2015) originally proposed the piecewise exponential models for dependent censoring, but did not use copulas. Consequently, the sub-density functions in their likelihood function require some numerical integrations of the joint density of T and U.

4.5 Semi-parametric Models

4.5.1 The Transformation Model

Chen (2010) considered a semi-parametric transformation model defined as

$$S_T(t|\mathbf{x}_{1i}) = \exp[-G_1\{\Lambda_0(t)e^{\beta_1'\mathbf{x}_{1i}}\}], \quad S_U(u|\mathbf{x}_{2i}) = \exp[-G_2\{\Gamma_0(u)e^{\beta_2'\mathbf{x}_{2i}}\}],$$

where β_j are regression coefficients, and $G_j(\cdot)$ is a known and nonnegative increasing function such that $G_j(0) = 0$, $G_j(\infty) = \infty$, and $g_j(t) \equiv dG_j(t)/dt > 0$ for $j = 1$ and 2; Λ_0 and Γ_0 are unknown increasing functions. No distributional assumptions are imposed on Λ_0 and Γ_0. The linear transformation $G_j(t) = t$ corresponds to the Cox model.

Under the semi-parametric transformation model, the cause-specific hazard functions are

$$h_T^{\#}(t|\mathbf{x}_i) = \lambda_0(t)e^{\boldsymbol{\beta}_1'\mathbf{x}_{1i}}\eta_{1i}(t;\boldsymbol{\beta}_1,\boldsymbol{\beta}_2,\Lambda_0,\Gamma_0|\theta), \quad h_U^{\#}(t|\mathbf{x}_i) = \gamma_0(t)e^{\boldsymbol{\beta}_2'\mathbf{x}_{2i}}\eta_{2i}(t;\boldsymbol{\beta}_1,\boldsymbol{\beta}_2,\Lambda_0,\Gamma_0|\theta),$$

where $\lambda_0(t) = d\Lambda_0(t)/dt$, $\gamma_0(t) = d\Gamma_0(t)/dt$,

$$\eta_{1i}(t;\boldsymbol{\beta}_1,\boldsymbol{\beta}_2,\Lambda_0,\Gamma_0|\theta) = g_1\{\Lambda_0(t)e^{\boldsymbol{\beta}_1'\mathbf{x}_{1i}}\}S_T(t|\mathbf{x}_{1i})D_{\theta,1}[S_T(t|\mathbf{x}_{1i}),S_U(t|\mathbf{x}_{2i})],$$
$$\eta_{2i}(t;\boldsymbol{\beta}_1,\boldsymbol{\beta}_2,\Lambda_0,\Gamma_0|\theta) = g_2\{\Gamma_0(t)e^{\boldsymbol{\beta}_2'\mathbf{x}_{2i}}\}S_U(t|\mathbf{x}_{2i})D_{\theta,2}[S_T(t|\mathbf{x}_{1i}),S_U(t|\mathbf{x}_{2i})],$$

$$D_{\theta,1}(u,v) = \frac{\partial C_\theta(u,v)/\partial u}{C_\theta(u,v)}, \quad D_{\theta,2}(u,v) = \frac{\partial C_\theta(u,v)/\partial v}{C_\theta(u,v)}.$$

Under the independence copula $C_\theta(u,v) = uv$, the cause-specific hazard functions are equal to the marginal hazards:

$$h_T^{\#}(t|\mathbf{x}_i) = \lambda_0(t)e^{\boldsymbol{\beta}_1'\mathbf{x}_{1i}}g_1\{\Lambda_0(t)e^{\boldsymbol{\beta}_1'\mathbf{x}_{1i}}\}, \quad h_U^{\#}(t|\mathbf{x}_i) = \gamma_0(t)e^{\boldsymbol{\beta}_2'\mathbf{x}_{2i}}g_2\{\Gamma_0(t)e^{\boldsymbol{\beta}_2'\mathbf{x}_{2i}}\}.$$

To obtain the MLE of $(\boldsymbol{\beta}_1,\boldsymbol{\beta}_2,\Lambda_0,\Gamma_0)$, we treat Λ_0 and Γ_0 as increasing step functions that have jumps sizes $d\Lambda_0(t_i) = \Lambda_0(t_i) - \Lambda_0(t_i-)$ for $\delta_i = 1$ and $d\Gamma_0(t_i) = \Gamma_0(t_i) - \Gamma_0(t_i-)$ for $\delta_i = 0$. Putting the cause-specific hazard functions into Eq. (4.5) and replacing $\lambda_0(t_i)$ by $d\Lambda_0(t_i)$ and $\gamma_0(t_i)$ by $d\Gamma_0(t_i)$, we obtain the log-likelihood

$$\ell(\boldsymbol{\beta}_1,\boldsymbol{\beta}_2,\Lambda_0,\Gamma_0|\theta) = \sum_i \delta_i[\boldsymbol{\beta}_1'\mathbf{x}_{1i} + \log\eta_{1i}(t_i;\boldsymbol{\beta}_1,\boldsymbol{\beta}_2,\Lambda_0,\Gamma_0|\theta) + \log d\Lambda_0(t_i)]$$
$$+ \sum_i (1-\delta_i)[\boldsymbol{\beta}_2'\mathbf{x}_{2i} + \log\eta_{2i}(t_i;\boldsymbol{\beta}_1,\boldsymbol{\beta}_2,\Lambda_0,\Gamma_0|\theta) + \log d\Gamma_0(t_i)]$$
$$- \sum_i \Phi_\theta[S_T(t_i|\mathbf{x}_{1i}),S_U(t_i|\mathbf{x}_{2i})],$$

where $\Phi_\theta(u,v) = -\log C_\theta(u,v)$. Since the marginal distributions have a number of parameters to be estimated, the profile likelihood may not properly identify a suitable value of θ. Chen (2010) suggested a sensitivity analysis to examine the result under a few different values of θ, possibly selected by prior knowledge and expert opinion.

The approach of Chen (2010) reduces to Cox's partial likelihood approach (Cox 1972) under the independence copula and the linear transformation. Under these assumptions, the MLE $(\hat{\boldsymbol{\beta}}_1,\hat{\boldsymbol{\beta}}_2,\hat{\Lambda}_0,\hat{\Gamma}_0)$ is obtained by maximizing two functions

$$\ell_1(\boldsymbol{\beta}_1,\Lambda_0) = \sum_i \delta_i[\boldsymbol{\beta}_1'\mathbf{x}_{1i} + \log d\Lambda_0(t_i)] + \sum_i \log S_T(t_i|\mathbf{x}_{1i}),$$
$$\ell_2(\boldsymbol{\beta}_2,\Gamma_0) = \sum_i (1-\delta_i)[\boldsymbol{\beta}_2'\mathbf{x}_{2i} + \log d\Gamma_0(t_i)] + \sum_i \log S_U(t_i|\mathbf{x}_{2i}),$$

since $\ell(\boldsymbol{\beta}_1, \boldsymbol{\beta}_2, \Lambda_0, \Gamma_0) = \ell_1(\boldsymbol{\beta}_1, \Lambda_0) + \ell_2(\boldsymbol{\beta}_2, \Gamma_0)$. Then, the MLE $(\hat{\boldsymbol{\beta}}_1, \hat{\Lambda}_0)$ for $(\boldsymbol{\beta}_1, \Lambda_0)$ is the partial likelihood estimator $\hat{\boldsymbol{\beta}}_1$ and the Breslow estimator $\hat{\Lambda}_0$ (Chap. 2).

4.5.2 The Spline Model

Emura et al. (2017) considered a spline-based model defined as

$$S_T(t|\mathbf{x}_{1i}) = \exp\{-\Lambda_0(t)e^{\boldsymbol{\beta}_1'\mathbf{x}_{1i}}\}, \quad S_U(u|\mathbf{x}_{2i}) = \exp\{-\Gamma_0(u)e^{\boldsymbol{\beta}_2'\mathbf{x}_{2i}}\},$$

where $\boldsymbol{\beta}_j$ are regression coefficients, and the baseline hazard functions are modeled by

$$\frac{d}{dt}\Lambda_0(t) = \lambda_0(t) = \sum_{\ell=1}^{5} g_\ell M_\ell(t) = \mathbf{g}'\mathbf{M}(t), \quad \frac{d}{dt}\Gamma_0(t) = \gamma_0(t) = \sum_{\ell=1}^{5} h_\ell M_\ell(t) = \mathbf{h}'\mathbf{M}(t),$$

where $\mathbf{M}(t) = (M_1(t), \ldots, M_5(t))'$ are the cubic M-spline basis functions (Ramsay 1988). Here, $\mathbf{g}' = (g_1, \ldots, g_5)$ and $\mathbf{h}' = (h_1, \ldots, h_5)$ are unknown positive parameters. These five-parameter approximations give a good flexibility in estimation for real applications (Ramsay 1988) and are one of reasonable choices (Commenges and Jacqmin-Gadda 2015). Since the spline bases are easy to integrate, the baseline cumulative hazard functions are computed as $\Lambda_0(t) = \sum_{\ell=1}^{5} g_\ell I_\ell(t)$ and $\Gamma_0(t) = \sum_{\ell=1}^{5} h_\ell I_\ell(t)$, where $I_\ell(t)$ is the integration of $M_\ell(t)$, called the *I-spline* basis (Ramsay 1988).

The *joint.Cox* package (Emura 2018) offers functions *M.spline* () for computing $M_\ell(t)$ and *I.spline* () for $I_\ell(t)$. To compute these spline bases, one needs to specify the range of t. The package uses the range $t \in [\xi_1, \xi_3]$ for the equally spaced knots $\xi_1 < \xi_2 < \xi_3$, where $\xi_2 = (\xi_1 + \xi_3)/2$. A possible choice is $\xi_1 = \min_i(t_i)$ and $\xi_3 = \max_i(t_i)$. The expressions of $M_\ell(t)$ and $I_\ell(t)$ are given in Appendix A. Figure 4.1 displays the M- and I-spline basis functions with the knots $\xi_1 = 1$, $\xi_2 = 2$, and $\xi_3 = 3$.

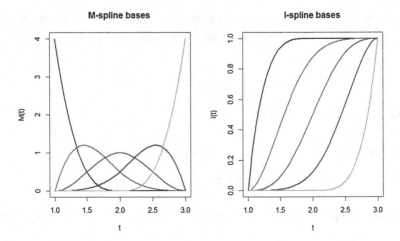

Fig. 4.1 M-spline basis functions (left-panel) and I-spline basis functions (right-panel) with knots $\xi_1 = 1$, $\xi_2 = 2$, and $\xi_3 = 3$

Under the spline model, the cause-specific hazard functions are

$$h_T^{\#}(t|\mathbf{x}_i) = \lambda_0(t)e^{\boldsymbol{\beta}_1'\mathbf{x}_{1i}}\eta_{1i}(t;\boldsymbol{\beta}_1,\boldsymbol{\beta}_2,\Lambda_0,\Gamma_0|\theta), \quad h_U^{\#}(t|\mathbf{x}_i) = \gamma_0(t)e^{\boldsymbol{\beta}_2'\mathbf{x}_{2i}}\eta_{2i}(t;\boldsymbol{\beta}_1,\boldsymbol{\beta}_2,\Lambda_0,\Gamma_0|\theta),$$

where

$$\eta_{1i}(t;\boldsymbol{\beta}_1,\boldsymbol{\beta}_2,\Lambda_0,\Gamma_0|\theta) = S_T(t|\mathbf{x}_{1i})D_{\theta,1}[S_T(t|\mathbf{x}_{1i}),S_U(t|\mathbf{x}_{2i})],$$
$$\eta_{2i}(t;\boldsymbol{\beta}_1,\boldsymbol{\beta}_2,\Lambda_0,\Gamma_0|\theta) = S_U(t|\mathbf{x}_{2i})D_{\theta,2}[S_T(t|\mathbf{x}_{1i}),S_U(t|\mathbf{x}_{2i})].$$

Putting these formulas into Eq. (4.5), we obtain the log-likelihood

$$\ell(\boldsymbol{\beta}_1,\boldsymbol{\beta}_2,\mathbf{g},\mathbf{h}|\theta) = \sum_i \delta_i[\boldsymbol{\beta}_1'\mathbf{x}_{1i} + \log\eta_{1i}(t_i;\boldsymbol{\beta}_1,\boldsymbol{\beta}_2,\Lambda_0,\Gamma_0|\theta) + \log\lambda_0(t_i)]$$
$$+ \sum_i (1-\delta_i)[\boldsymbol{\beta}_2'\mathbf{x}_{2i} + \log\eta_{2i}(t_i;\boldsymbol{\beta}_1,\boldsymbol{\beta}_2,\Lambda_0,\Gamma_0|\theta) + \log\gamma_0(t_i)]$$
$$- \sum_i \Phi_\theta[S_T(t_i|\mathbf{x}_{1i}),S_U(t_i|\mathbf{x}_{2i})].$$

The estimator of $(\boldsymbol{\beta}_1,\boldsymbol{\beta}_2,\mathbf{g},\mathbf{h})$ is obtained by maximizing the penalized log-likelihood

$$\ell(\boldsymbol{\beta}_1,\boldsymbol{\beta}_2,\mathbf{g},\mathbf{h}|\theta) - \kappa_1\int\ddot{\lambda}_0(t)^2dt - \kappa_2\int\ddot{\gamma}_0(t)^2dt,$$

where $\ddot{f}(t) = d^2f(t)/dt^2$, and (κ_1, κ_2) are given nonnegative values. The parameters (κ_1, κ_2) are called *smoothing parameters*, which control the degrees of penalties on the roughness of the two baseline hazard functions. It is shown in Appendix A that

$$\int_{\xi_1}^{\xi_3} \ddot{\lambda}_0(t)^2 dt = \mathbf{g}'\Omega\mathbf{g}, \qquad \int_{\xi_1}^{\xi_3} \ddot{\gamma}_0(t)^2 dt = \mathbf{h}'\Omega\mathbf{h},$$

$$\Omega = \frac{1}{\Delta^5} \begin{bmatrix} 192 & -132 & 24 & 12 & 0 \\ -132 & 96 & -24 & -12 & 12 \\ 24 & -24 & 24 & -24 & 24 \\ 12 & -12 & -24 & 96 & -132 \\ 0 & 12 & 24 & -132 & 192 \end{bmatrix},$$

where $\Delta = \xi_2 - \xi_1 = \xi_3 - \xi_2$. A naïve approach is to set $\kappa_1 = \kappa_2 = 0$ as in Shih and Emura (2018).

A more sophisticated approach is to choose (κ_1, κ_2) by optimizing a likelihood cross-validation (LCV) criterion (O' Sullivan 1988). Under the independence copula, the penalized log-likelihood is written as the sum of two marginal penalized log-likelihoods,

$$\left[\ell_1(\boldsymbol{\beta}_1, \Lambda_0) - \kappa_1 \int \ddot{\lambda}_0(t)^2 dt\right] + \left[\ell_2(\boldsymbol{\beta}_2, \Gamma_0) - \kappa_2 \int \ddot{\gamma}_0(t)^2 dt\right],$$

where

$$\ell_1(\boldsymbol{\beta}_1, \Lambda_0) = \sum_i \delta_i[\boldsymbol{\beta}_1'\mathbf{x}_{1i} + \log \lambda_0(t_i)] - \sum_i \Lambda_0(t_i)\exp(\boldsymbol{\beta}_1'\mathbf{x}_{1i}),$$

$$\ell_2(\boldsymbol{\beta}_2, \Gamma_0) = \sum_i (1 - \delta_i)[\boldsymbol{\beta}_2'\mathbf{x}_{2i} + \log \gamma_0(t_i)] - \sum_i \Gamma_0(t_i)\exp(\boldsymbol{\beta}_2'\mathbf{x}_{2i}).$$

We suggest choosing κ_1 and κ_2 based on the two marginal LCVs defined as

$$LCV_1 = \hat{\ell}_1 - \text{tr}\{\hat{H}_{PL1}^{-1}\hat{H}_1\}, \quad LCV_2 = \hat{\ell}_2 - \text{tr}\{\hat{H}_{PL2}^{-1}\hat{H}_2\},$$

where $\hat{\ell}_1$ and $\hat{\ell}_2$ are the log-likelihood values evaluated at their marginal penalized likelihood estimates, and $\hat{H}_{PL1}$ and $\hat{H}_{PL2}$ are the converged Hessian matrices for the marginal penalized likelihood estimations, $\hat{H}_1$ and $\hat{H}_2$ are the converged Hessian matrices for the marginal log-likelihoods such that

$$\hat{H}_1 = \hat{H}_{PL1} + 2\kappa_1 \begin{bmatrix} O_{p_1 \times p_1} & O_{p_1 \times 5} \\ O_{5 \times p_1} & \Omega \end{bmatrix}, \quad \hat{H}_2 = \hat{H}_{PL2} + 2\kappa_2 \begin{bmatrix} O_{p_2 \times p_2} & O_{p_2 \times 5} \\ O_{5 \times p_2} & \Omega \end{bmatrix},$$

where O is a zero matrix and p_j is the dimension of $\boldsymbol{\beta}_j$ for $j = 1$ and 2. The values of (κ_1, κ_2) are obtained by maximizing LCV_1 for κ_1 and LCV_2 for κ_2, separately. One may apply the R function *splineCox.reg* in the *joint.Cox* R package to find the optimal value of κ_1 (or κ_2).

References

Amini M, Jabbari H, Mohtashami Borzadaran GR (2011) Aspects of dependence in generalized Farlie-Gumbel-Morgenstern distributions. Commun Stat Simul Comput 40(8):1192–1205

Braekers R, Veraverbeke N (2005) A copula-graphic estimator for the conditional survival function under dependent censoring. Can J Stat 33:429–447

Chaieb LL, Rivest LP, Abdous B (2006) Estimating survival under a dependent truncation. Biometrika 93(3):655–669

Chen YH (2010) Semiparametric marginal regression analysis for dependent competing risks under an assumed copula. J R Stat Soc Ser B Stat Methodol 72:235–251

Collett D (2015) Modelling survival data in medical research, 3rd edn. CRC Press, London

Commenges D, Jacqmin-Gadda H (2015) Dynamical biostatistical models. CRC Press, London

Cox DR (1972) Regression models and life-tables (with discussion). J R Stat Soc Ser B Stat Methodol 34:187–220

de Uña-Álvarez J, Veraverbeke N (2013) Generalized copula-graphic estimator. TEST 22(2):343–360

de Uña-Álvarez J, Veraverbeke N (2017) Copula-graphic estimation with left-truncated and right-censored data. Statistics 51(2):387–403

Domma F, Giordano S (2013) A copula-based approach to account for dependence in stress-strength models. Stat Pap 54(3):807–826

Emura T, Chen YH (2016) Gene selection for survival data under dependent censoring, a copula-based approach. Stat Methods Med Res 25(6):2840–2857

Emura T, Murotani K (2015) An algorithm for estimating survival under a copula-based dependent truncation model. TEST 24(4):734–751

Emura T, Michimae H (2017) A copula-based inference to piecewise exponential models under dependent censoring, with application to time to metamorphosis of salamander larvae. Environ Ecol Stat 24(1):151–173

Emura T, Nakatochi M, Murotani K, Rondeau V (2017) A joint frailty-copula model between tumour progression and death for meta-analysis. Stat Methods Med Res 26(6):2649–2666

Emura T (2018) joint.Cox: penalized likelihood estimation and dynamic prediction under the joint frailty-copula models between tumour progression and death for meta-analysis, CRAN

Emura T, Chen HY, Matsui S, Chen YH (2018) compound.Cox: univariate feature selection and compound covariate for predicting survival, CRAN

Escarela G, Carrière JF (2003) Fitting competing risks with an assumed copula. Stat Methods Med Res 12(4):333–349

Heckman JJ, Honore BE (1989) The identifiability of the competing risks models. Biometrika 76:325–330

Hu YH, Emura T (2015) Maximum likelihood estimation for a special exponential family under random double-truncation. Comput Stat 30(4):1199–1229

Moradian H, Denis Larocque D, Bellavance F (2017). Survival forests for data with dependent censoring. Stat Methods Med Res, https://doi.org/10.1177/0962280217727314

Nelsen RB (2006) An introduction to copulas, 2nd edn. Springer, New York

O' Sullivan F (1988) Fast computation of fully automated log-density and log-hazard estimation. SIAM J Sci Stat Comput 9:363–379

Ramsay J (1988) Monotone regression spline in action. Stat Sci 3:425–461

Rivest LP, Wells MT (2001) A martingale approach to the copula-graphic estimator for the survival function under dependent censoring. J Multivar Anal 79:138–155

Shih JH, Emura T (2016) Bivariate dependence measures and bivariate competing risks models under the generalized FGM copula. Stat Pap, https://doi.org/10.1007/s00362-016-0865-5

Shih JH, Lee W, Sun LH, Emura T (2018) Fitting competing risks data to bivariate Pareto models. Commun Stat Theory, https://doi.org/10.1080/03610926.2018.1425450

Shih JH, Emura T (2018) Likelihood-based inference for bivariate latent failure time models with competing risks under the generalized FGM copula. Comput Stat, https://doi.org/10.1007/s00180-018-0804-0

Shih JH (2018) GFGM.copula: generalized Farlie-Gumbel-Morgenstern copula, CRAN

Shih JH and Lee W (2018) Bivariate.Pareto: bivariate Pareto models, CRAN

Staplin ND (2012) Informative censoring in transplantation statistics. Doctoral Thesis, University of Southampton, School of Mathematics

Staplin ND, Kimber AC, Collett D, Roderick PJ (2015) Dependent censoring in piecewise exponential survival models. Stat Methods Med Res 24(3):325–341

Tsiatis A (1975) A nonidentifiability aspect of the problem of competing risks. Proc Natl Acad Sci 72(1):20–22

Zheng M, Klein JP (1995) Estimates of marginal survival for dependent competing risks based on an assumed copula. Biometrika 82(1):127–138

Chapter 5
Gene Selection and Survival Prediction Under Dependent Censoring

Abstract To select genes that are predictive of survival, univariate selection based on the Cox model has been routinely employed in biomedical research. However, this conventional approach relies on the independent censoring assumption, which is often an unrealistic assumption in many biomedical applications. We introduce an alternative approach to selecting genes by utilizing copulas to account for the effect of dependent censoring. We also introduce a method to construct a predictor based on the selected genes to predict patient survival. We use the non-small-cell lung cancer data to demonstrate the copula-based procedure for selecting genes, developing a predictor, and validating the predictor. We provide detailed instructions to implement the proposed statistical methods and to reproduce the real data analyses through the *compound.Cox* R package.

Keywords Clayton's copula · Competing risk · Compound covariate Copula-graphic estimator · Cox regression · C-index · Gene expression Overall survival · Univariate selection

5.1 Introduction

Recent years have witnessed a rapid increase in the use of genetic covariates to build survival prediction models in biomedical research. Accurate prediction of survival is often possible by incorporating genetic covariates into prediction models, as reported in breast cancer (Jenssen et al. 2002; Sabatier et al. 2011; Zhao et al. 2011), diffuse large-B-cell lymphoma (Lossos et al. 2004; Alizadeh et al. 2011), lung cancer (Beer et al. 2002; Chen et al. 2007; Shedden et al. 2008), ovarian cancer (Popple et al. 2012; Yoshihara et al. 2010, 2012; Waldron et al. 2014), and other cancers. Evaluating predictive accuracy of the survival prediction models has been a challenging area of research due to the high-dimensionality of genes (Michiels et al. 2005; Schumacher et al. 2007; Bøvelstad et al. 2007, 2009; Witten and Tibshirani 2010; Zhao et al. 2014; Emura et al. 2017).

© The Author(s) 2018   57
T. Emura and Y.-H. Chen, *Analysis of Survival Data with Dependent Censoring*,
JSS Research Series in Statistics, https://doi.org/10.1007/978-981-10-7164-5_5

To overcome the difficulty of handling the high-dimensional genetic covariates, one often needs to obtain a small fraction of genes that are predictive of survival. The traditional approach, called *univariate selection*, is a forward variable selection method according to univariate association between each gene and survival, where the association is measured through univariate Cox regression. A predictor constructed from the selected genes has been shown to be useful for survival prediction (Beer et al. 2002; Wang et al. 2005; Matsui 2006; Chen et al. 2007; Matsui et al. 2012; Emura et al. 2017).

It is well known that Cox regression relies on the independent censoring assumption. From our discussions in Chap. 3, this assumption seems unrealistic in univariate Cox regression, where many covariates are omitted. If the independent censoring assumption is violated, univariate Cox regression may not correctly capture the effect of each gene and thus may fail to select useful genes. Accordingly, the resultant predictor based on the selected genes may have a reduced ability to predict survival.

Emura and Chen (2016) introduced a copula-based method for performing gene selection. With this method, dependence between survival and censoring times is modeled via a copula, whereby relaxing the independent censoring assumption. In the subsequent discussions, we revisit their method by providing more detailed developments than the original paper. We have made the lung cancer data publicly available in the *compound.Cox* R package (Emura et al. 2018) to enhance reproducibility.

The chapter is organized as follows. Section 5.2 reviews the conventional univariate selection. Sections 5.3–5.5 introduce the copula-based method of Emura and Chen (2016). Section 5.6 includes the analysis of the non-small-cell lung cancer data for illustration. Section 5.7 provides discussions.

5.2 Univariate Selection

Univariate selection is the traditional method for selecting a subset of genes that is predictive of survival. As the initial step, one fits the univariate Cox model for each gene, one-by-one. Then, one selects a subset of genes that are univariately associated with survival. Finally, one builds a multi-gene predictor using the subset of genes for purpose of survival prediction. The predictor is usually a weighted sum of gene expressions whose weights reflect the degree of association.

Let $\mathbf{x} = (x_1, \ldots, x_p)'$ be a p-dimensional vector of gene expressions, where the dimension p can be large. Let T be survival time having the hazard function $h(t|\mathbf{x}) = \Pr(t \leq T < t + dt \,|T \geq t, \, \mathbf{x} \,)/dt$. It is well known that the multivariate Cox model $h(t|\mathbf{x}) = h_0(t) \exp(\boldsymbol{\beta}'\mathbf{x})$ does not yield proper estimates of $\boldsymbol{\beta}$ when p is very large (Witten and Tibshirani 2010).

In biomedical research, the univariate Cox regression analysis is the traditional strategy to deal with the large number of covariates (e.g., Beer et al. 2002; Chen et al. 2007). Let $h(t|x_j) = \Pr(t \leq T < t + dt \,|T \geq t, \, x_j \,)/dt$ be the hazard function given the jth gene. The univariate Cox model is specified as $h_j(t|x_j) = h_{0j}(t)\exp(\beta_j x_j)$ for each gene $j = 1, \ldots, p$. The primary objective of using the univariate Cox model is to perform univariate selection as follows: For each $j = 1, \ldots, p$, the null hypothesis $H_0 : \beta_j = 0$ is examined by the Wald test (or score test) under the univariate Cox model. Then one picks out a subset of genes that have low P-values from the tests. The genes with low P-values are then selected for further analysis.

After genes are selected, they are used to build a prediction scheme for survival. In medical studies, it is a common practice to re-fit a multivariate Cox regression model based on the selected genes (e.g., Lossos et al. 2004). However, we have reservations about this commonly used strategy due to the poor predictive performance observed in many papers (e.g., Bøvelstad et al. 2007; van Wieringen et al. 2009). Alternatively, we suggest using Tukey's compound covariate predictor (Tukey 1993) that combines the results of univariate analyses without going through a multivariate analysis. The compound covariate has been successfully employed in many medical studies (e.g., Beer et al. 2002; Wang et al. 2005; Chen et al. 2007) and biostatistical studies (Matsui 2006; Matsui et al. 2012; Emura et al. 2012, 2017).

The two major assumptions of univariate selection are the correctness of the univariate Cox model and the independent censoring assumption. The violation of these assumptions yields bias in estimating the true effect of genes. Emura and Chen (2016) argued that the independence of censoring is a more crucial assumption than the correctness of the univariate Cox model. The bias due to dependent censoring gets large if either the degree of dependence or the percentage of censoring increases (see Sect. 3.5). In the following sections, we shall introduce a copula-based univariate selection method that copes with the problem of dependent censoring.

5.3 Copula-Based Univariate Cox Regression

Let T be survival time, U be censoring time, and $\mathbf{x} = (x_1, \ldots, x_p)'$ be gene expressions. The joint distribution of T and U can have an arbitrary dependence pattern for any given x_j. Sklar's theorem (Sklar 1959; Nelsen 2006) guarantees that the joint survival function is expressed as

$$\Pr(T > t, U > u|x_j) = C_j\{\Pr(T > t|x_j), \Pr(U > u|x_j)\}, \quad j = 1, \ldots, p,$$

where C_j is a copula. The *independent censoring assumption* corresponds to $C_j(u, v) = uv$ for $j = 1, \ldots, p$, namely,

$$\Pr(T > t, U > u|x_j) = \Pr(T > t|x_j) \times \Pr(U > u|x_j), \quad j = 1, \ldots, p. \quad (5.1)$$

This is clearly a strong assumption (Chap. 3).

To relax the independent censoring assumption, Emura and Chen (2016) suggested a one-parameter copula model

$$\Pr(\,T > t\,,\; U > u|x_j\,) = C_\alpha\{\,\Pr(\,T > t\,|x_j\,),\; \Pr(\,U > u|x_j\,)\,\}, \quad j = 1,\, \ldots,\, p. \quad (5.2)$$

Since the same copula C is assumed for every j, this assumption may still be strong. Nevertheless, the copula relaxes the independent censoring assumption (5.1) by allowing a dependence parameter α to be flexibly chosen by users. One example is the Clayton copula

$$C_\alpha(\,u,\,v\,) = (\,u^{-\alpha} + v^{-\alpha} - 1\,)^{-1/\alpha}, \qquad \alpha > 0,$$

where the parameter α is related to Kendall's tau through $\tau = \alpha/(\alpha + 2)$. The copula model (5.2) reduces to the independent censoring model (5.1) by letting $\alpha \to 0$.

For marginal distributions, Emura and Chen (2016) assumed the Cox models

$$\Pr(\,T > t\,|x_j\,) = \exp\{\,-\Lambda_{0j}(t)e^{\beta_j x_j}\,\}, \quad \Pr(\,U > u\,|x_j\,) = \exp\{\,-\Gamma_{0j}(u)e^{\gamma_j x_j}\,\}, \tag{5.3}$$

where β_j and γ_j are regression coefficients and Λ_{0j} and Γ_{0j} are baseline cumulative hazard functions.

For purpose of gene selection, the target parameter is β_j that is the univariate effect of the jth gene on survival. Other parameters (γ_j, Λ_{0j}, Γ_{0j}) are nuisance. Under the independent censoring model (5.1), one can use the partial likelihood to estimate for β_j while ignoring the nuisance parameters. However, under the copula model (5.2), the partial likelihood estimator gives an inconsistent estimate of β_j (Chap. 3).

The full likelihood is necessary to consistently estimate (β_j, γ_j, Λ_{0j}, Γ_{0j}) under the copula model (5.2) and the Cox models (5.3). Define notations

$$D_{\alpha,1}(u,\,v) = \frac{\partial C_\alpha(u,\,v)/\partial u}{C_\alpha(u,\,v)} = -\frac{\partial \Phi_\alpha(u,\,v)}{\partial u},$$

$$D_{\alpha,2}(u,\,v) = \frac{\partial C_\alpha(u,\,v)/\partial v}{C_\alpha(u,\,v)} = -\frac{\partial \Phi_\alpha(u,\,v)}{\partial v},$$

where $\Phi_\alpha(u,v) = -\log C_\alpha(u,v)$. Observed data are denoted as $\{(t_i, \delta_i, x_{ij}), i = 1, \ldots, n\}$, where $t_i = \min(T_i, U_i)$ and $\delta_i = \mathbf{I}(T_i \le U_i)$, where $\mathbf{I}(\cdot)$ is the indicator function. As in Chen (2010), we treat Λ_{0j} and Γ_{0j} as increasing step functions that have jumps sizes $d\Lambda_{0j}(t_i) = \Lambda_{0j}(t_i) - \Lambda_{0j}(t_i - dt)$ for $\delta_i = 1$ and $d\Gamma_{0j}(t_i) = \Gamma_{0j}(t_i) - \Gamma_{0j}(t_i - dt)$ for $\delta_i = 0$. For any given α, the log-likelihood is defined as

$$\ell(\beta_j,\, \gamma_j,\, \Lambda_{0j},\, \Gamma_{0j}|\alpha) = \sum_i \delta_i[\,\beta_j x_{ij} + \log \eta_{1ij}(t_i;\, \beta_j,\, \gamma_j,\, \Lambda_{0j},\, \Gamma_{0j}|\alpha) + \log d\Lambda_{0j}(t_i)\,]$$

$$+ \sum_i (1 - \delta_i)[\,\gamma_j x_{ij} + \log \eta_{2ij}(t_i;\, \beta_j,\, \gamma_j,\, \Lambda_{0j},\, \Gamma_{0j}|\alpha) + \log d\Gamma_{0j}(t_i)\,]$$

$$- \sum_i \Phi_\alpha[\,\exp\{\,-\Lambda_{0j}(t_i)e^{\beta_j x_{ij}}\,\},\; \exp\{\,-\Gamma_{0j}(t_i)e^{\gamma_j x_{ij}}\,\}\,],$$

$$\tag{5.4}$$

where,

$$\eta_{1ij}(t; \beta_j, \gamma_j, \Lambda_{0j}, \Gamma_{0j}|\alpha) = \exp\{-\Lambda_{0j}(t)e^{\beta_j x_{ij}}\}D_{\alpha,1}[\exp\{-\Lambda_{0j}(t)e^{\beta_j x_{ij}}\}, \exp\{-\Gamma_{0j}(t)e^{\gamma_j x_{ij}}\}],$$
$$\eta_{2ij}(t; \beta_j, \gamma_j, \Lambda_{0j}, \Gamma_{0j}|\alpha) = \exp\{-\Gamma_{0j}(t)e^{\gamma_j x_{ij}}\}D_{\alpha,2}[\exp\{-\Lambda_{0j}(t)e^{\beta_j x_{ij}}\}, \exp\{-\Gamma_{0j}(t)e^{\gamma_j x_{ij}}\}].$$

The maximizer of Eq. (5.4) given α is denoted as $(\hat{\beta}_j(\alpha), \hat{\gamma}_j(\alpha), \hat{\Lambda}_{0j}(\alpha), \hat{\Gamma}_{0j}(\alpha))$. The standard error $SE\{\hat{\beta}_j(\alpha)\}$ is computed from the information matrix (Chen 2010).

The log-likelihood in Eq. (5.4) can be easily computed under the Clayton copula. It can be shown that $\Phi_\alpha(u, v) = \alpha^{-1}\log(u^{-\alpha} + v^{-\alpha} - 1)$, $D_{\alpha,1}(u, v) = u^{-\alpha-1}(u^{-\alpha} + v^{-\alpha} - 1)^{-1}$, and $D_{\alpha,2}(u, v) = u^{-\alpha-1}(u^{-\alpha} + v^{-\alpha} - 1)^{-1}$. Hence,

$$\eta_{1ij}(t; \beta_j, \gamma_j, \Lambda_{0j}, \Gamma_{0j}|\alpha) = \frac{[\exp\{-\Lambda_{0j}(t)e^{\beta_j x_{ij}}\}]^{-\alpha}}{[\exp\{-\Lambda_{0j}(t)e^{\beta_j x_{ij}}\}]^{-\alpha} + [\exp\{-\Gamma_{0j}(t)e^{\gamma_j x_{ij}}\}]^{-\alpha} - 1},$$
$$\eta_{2ij}(t; \beta_j, \gamma_j, \Lambda_{0j}, \Gamma_{0j}|\alpha) = \frac{[\exp\{-\Gamma_{0j}(t)e^{\gamma_j x_{ij}}\}]^{-\alpha}}{[\exp\{-\Lambda_{0j}(t)e^{\beta_j x_{ij}}\}]^{-\alpha} + [\exp\{-\Gamma_{0j}(t)e^{\gamma_j x_{ij}}\}]^{-\alpha} - 1}.$$

One can apply these formulas to Eq. (5.4) to calculate the log-likelihood function and maximize it by optimization algorithms.

We implemented the computation of $\hat{\beta}_j(\alpha)$ and $SE\{\hat{\beta}_j(\alpha)\}$ in the *compound.Cox* R package (Emura et al. 2018). In the package, the maximization of Eq. (5.4) is performed by the *nlm* function after the log-transformations $\log d\Lambda_{0j}(t_i)$ and $\log d\Gamma_{0j}(t_i)$. The package uses the initial values $\beta_j = \gamma_j = 0$ and $d\Lambda_{0j}(t_i) = d\Gamma_{0j}(t_i) = 1/n$.

Technical remarks: Theoretically, if $\alpha \downarrow 0$, $\hat{\beta}_j(\alpha)$ approaches to the partial likelihood estimate of β_j. Numerically, however, the value α too close to zero makes the likelihood optimization unstable. Hence, we set $\hat{\beta}_j(\alpha) = \hat{\beta}_j(0.01)$ for $0 \leq \alpha < 0.01$ in the package. The value of $\hat{\beta}_j(\alpha) = \hat{\beta}_j(0.01)$ is almost the same as the partial likelihood estimate.

5.4 Copula-Based Univariate Selection

One can use the copula-based method in Sect. 5.3 to perform univariate selection adjusted for the effect of dependent censoring. The P-value for testing the null hypothesis $H_0 : \beta_j = 0$ is computed by the Wald test based on a Z-statistic $\hat{\beta}_j(\alpha)/SE\{\hat{\beta}_j(\alpha)\}$. One can select a subset of genes according to the P-values. With $\alpha \approx 0$ in the Clayton copula, one has $C(u, v) \approx uv$. Hence, the resultant test is approximately equal to the Wald test under univariate Cox regression. In this sense, the copula-based test is a generalization of the conventional univariate selection.

For a future subject with a covariate vector $\mathbf{x} = (x_1, \ldots, x_p)'$, survival prediction can be made by the prognostic index (PI) defined as $\hat{\boldsymbol{\beta}}(\alpha)'\mathbf{x}$, where $\hat{\boldsymbol{\beta}}(\alpha)' = (\hat{\beta}_1(\alpha), \cdots, \hat{\beta}_p(\alpha))$. The PI is a weighted sum of genes whose weights reflect the degree of univariate association. If $\alpha = 0$, one obtains PI $= \hat{\boldsymbol{\beta}}(0)'\mathbf{x}$ which is equal to the *compound covariate* based on univariate Cox regression under the independent censoring assumption (Matsui 2006; Emura et al. 2012).

5.5 Choosing the Copula Parameter by the *C*-Index

Estimation of the copula parameter α is inherently difficult due to the non-identifiability of competing risks data (Tsiatis 1975). An estimator maximizing the profile log-likelihood for α based on Eq. (5.4) typically shows very large sampling variation (Chen 2010). In our experience, the profile likelihood often has a peak at extreme values; for instance, either $\alpha \approx 0$ or $\alpha \approx \infty$ under the Clayton copula. These undesirable properties make the likelihood-based strategy less useful.

Following Emura and Chen (2016), we introduce a prediction-based strategy for choosing α. A widely used predictive measure is a cross-validated partial likelihood (Verveij and van Houwelingen 1993). Unfortunately, the partial likelihood is not a valid likelihood under dependent censoring.

A more plausible predictive measure under dependent censoring is Harrell's *c*-index (Harrell et al. 1982). The interpretation of the *c*-index does not depend on a specific model. We adopt a cross-validated version of the *c*-index defined as follows.

We calculate the *c*-index based on a K-fold cross-validation. We first divide n patients into K groups of approximately equal sample sizes. This process can be specified by a function $\kappa : \{1, \ldots, n\} \mapsto \{1, \ldots K\}$ indicating the group to which each patient is allocated (Hastie et al. 2009). For each patient i, define the PI:

$$\mathrm{PI}_i(\alpha) = \hat{\boldsymbol{\beta}}'_{-\kappa(i)}(\alpha)\mathbf{x}_i = \hat{\beta}_{1,-\kappa(i)}(\alpha)x_{i1} + \cdots + \hat{\beta}_{p,-\kappa(i)}(\alpha)x_{ip},$$

where $\hat{\beta}_{j,-\kappa(i)}(\alpha)$ is obtained based on Eq. (5.4) with the $\kappa(i)$th group of patients removed. In this way, $\mathrm{PI}_i(\alpha)$ is a predictor of the survival outcome (t_i, δ_i) for the patient i. We define the cross-validated *c*-index:

$$CV(\alpha) = \frac{\sum_{i<j} \{ \mathbf{I}(t_i < t_j)\mathbf{I}(\mathrm{PI}_i(\alpha) > \mathrm{PI}_j(\alpha))\delta_i + \mathbf{I}(t_j < t_i)\mathbf{I}(\mathrm{PI}_j(\alpha) > \mathrm{PI}_i(\alpha))\delta_j \}}{\sum_{i<j} \{ \mathbf{I}(t_i < t_j)\delta_i + \mathbf{I}(t_j < t_i)\delta_j \}}.$$

Finally, we define $\hat{\alpha}$ that maximizes $CV(\alpha)$. We recommend $K = 5$ that is often used when n or p is large.

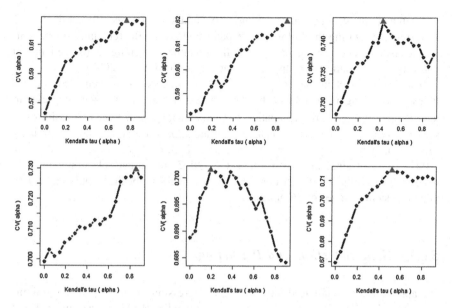

Fig. 5.1 Six replications of the cross-validated *c*-index $CV(\alpha)$. The maximum of $CV(\alpha)$ is signified as a triangle (in red color)

It is computationally demanding to obtain a high-dimensional vector $\hat{\beta}_{-\kappa(i)}(\alpha)$ for every group $\kappa(i)$. To release the computational cost, we suggest reducing the number p by using the initial univariate selection under $\alpha = 0$, e.g., based on P-value <0.2. The technique shall be applied to the subsequent data analysis.

A graphical diagnostic plot for $CV(\alpha)$ is informative to see how the proposed method of choosing $\hat{\alpha}$ works. We suggest using a grid search to find the approximate value of $\hat{\alpha}$ and plot the values of $CV(\alpha)$ against the grids. Figure 5.1 shows the plots of $CV(\alpha)$ with simulated data under our previously considered setting (Case 2 of Table 2 in Emura and Chen 2016). The figure shows that $CV(\hat{\alpha})$ is noticeably larger than $CV(0)$. This suggest that $\mathrm{PI}_i(\hat{\alpha})$ has better ability to predict survival than $\mathrm{PI}_i(0)$ does.

5.6   Lung Cancer Data Analysis

We analyze the survival data on the non-small-cell lung cancer patients of Chen et al. (2007). The data analysis was performed previously by Emura and Chen (2016) using the copula-based methods. Here, we update the analysis based on the data available in the *compound.Cox* R package, providing more detailed explanations than the previous one. In addition, this demonstration allows researchers to reproduce all the results easily through R.

In the lung cancer data, the primary endpoint is overall survival, i.e., time-to-death. During the follow-up, 38 patients died and the remaining 87 patients were censored. The 125 patients were split into either a training set (63 patients) or a testing set (62 patients) in the same manner as Chen et al. (2007).

The *Lung* object in the *compound.Cox* R package contains censored survival times t, censoring indicators δ_i, training/testing indicators, and gene expressions $\mathbf{x}_i = (x_{i1}, \ldots, x_{ip})'$ for the 125 patients. Available are $p = 97$ gene expressions that satisfy P-value <0.20 under the usual univariate selection performed on the training set. All the gene expressions were coded as 1, 2, 3, or 4 according to Chen et al. (2007). In the original analysis of Chen et al. (2007), univariate selection yielded 16 genes with P-value <0.05. In our analysis, we shall apply the copula-based univariate selection to select 16 genes.

5.6.1 Gene Selection and Prediction

We applied the copula-based univariate Cox regression to the 63 patients (training set) by using the R codes available in Appendix B. Here, we used $K = 5$ cross-validation for examining the diagnostic plot of $CV(\alpha)$. The outputs are shown below:

```
> res
$beta
VHL            IHPK1         HMMR         CMKOR1       PLAU
-0.093375981  -0.408433517  0.130353170  0.098116123  0.241605149
 :

$SE
VHL        IHPK1      HMMR       CMKOR1     PLAU
0.1769419  0.1686817  0.1635025  0.1913140  0.3552096
 :

$Z
VHL          IHPK1        HMMR         CMKOR1       PLAU
-0.52772110  -2.42132730  0.79725501   0.51285397   0.68017631
 :

$P
VHL            IHPK1         HMMR          CMKOR1        PLAU
0.5976929269  0.0154639470  0.4253029451  0.6080534771  0.4963928296
 :

$alpha
[1] 18

$c_index
[1] 0.6312719
```

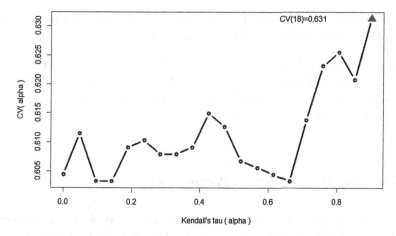

Fig. 5.2 Plot of $CV(\alpha)$ (the cross-validated c-index) based on the lung cancer data. The value of $CV(\alpha)$ is maximized at $\alpha = 18$ (Kendall's tau = 0.90)

Here, $beta = \hat{\beta}_j(\hat{\alpha})$, $SE = SE\{\hat{\beta}_j(\hat{\alpha})\}$, $Z = \hat{\beta}_j(\hat{\alpha})/SE\{\hat{\beta}_j(\hat{\alpha})\}$, and $P is the P-value for each $j = 1, \ldots, 97$. Also, $alpha = \hat{\alpha}$ and $c\_index = CV(\hat{\alpha})$.

Figure 5.2 displays the diagnostic plot of the cross-validated c-index $CV(\alpha)$ calculated on the 63 patients (training set). The c-index is maximized at the copula parameter $\hat{\alpha} = 18$ (Kendall's tau = 0.90). This implies a possible gain in prediction accuracy by using the Clayton copula for dependent censoring.

We selected the 16 genes among the 97 genes according to the P-values. The outputs are shown below:

	Coef	P.value
MMP16	0.51	0.0003
ZNF264	0.51	0.0004
HGF	0.50	0.0010
HCK	-0.49	0.0012
NF1	0.47	0.0016
ERBB3	0.46	0.0016
NR2F6	0.57	0.0030
AXL	0.77	0.0034
CDC23	0.51	0.0051
DLG2	0.92	0.0054
IGF2	-0.34	0.0081
RBBP6	0.54	0.0082
COX11	0.51	0.0116
DUSP6	0.40	0.0122
ENG	-0.37	0.0140
IHPK1	-0.41	0.0155

The resultant PI is defined as $\mathrm{PI} = \hat{\beta}_j(\hat{\alpha})x_1 + \cdots + \hat{\beta}_{16}(\hat{\alpha})x_{16}$, where $(x_1, \ldots, x_{16})$ are gene expressions of the 16 genes. Accordingly,

$$
\begin{aligned}
\mathrm{PI} = \; & (0.51 \times \mathrm{MMP16}) + (0.51 \times \mathrm{ZNF264}) + (0.50 \times \mathrm{HGF}) + (-0.49 \times \mathrm{HCK}) + (0.47 \times \mathrm{NF1}) \\
& + (0.46 \times \mathrm{ERBB3}) + (0.57 \times \mathrm{NR2F6}) + (0.77 \times \mathrm{AXL}) + (0.51 \times \mathrm{CDC23}) + (0.92 \times \mathrm{DLG2}) \\
& + (-0.34 \times \mathrm{IGF2}) + (0.54 \times \mathrm{RBBP6}) + (0.51 \times \mathrm{COX11}) + (0.40 \times \mathrm{DUSP6}) + (-0.37 \times \mathrm{ENG}) \\
& + (-0.41 \times \mathrm{IHPK1}).
\end{aligned}
$$

5.6.2   Assessing Prediction Performance

To validate the ability of the PI for predicting overall survival, we separate the 62 testing patients into two groups of equal sizes: 31 good prognosis patients with low PIs and 31 poor prognosis patients with high PIs. We then calculate the two survival curves for each group (Fig. 5.3).

The prediction performance of the PI can be measured by the difference between the two survival curves in Fig. 5.3. The two survival curves were calculated by the *copula-graphic estimator* (Rivest and Wells 2001) that adjusts for the effect of dependent censoring with the Clayton copula at $\hat{\alpha} = 18$ (Kendall's tau = 0.90). This approach may be better than the conventional log-rank test to measure the difference between two Kaplan–Meier estimators that are biased under dependent censoring.

Under the Clayton copula model, the copula-graphic (CG) estimator (Chap. 4) is defined as

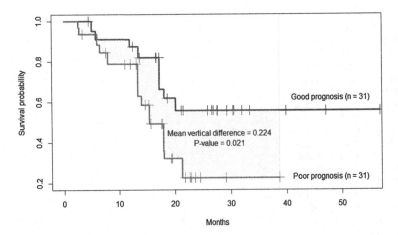

Fig. 5.3 Survival curves for the good and poor prognosis groups. The good (or poor) group is determined by the low (or high) values of the PI. Censored patients are indicated as the mark "+"

$$\hat{S}^{CG}(t) = \left[1 + \sum_{t_i \leq t, \, \delta_i = 1} \left\{ \left(\frac{n_i - 1}{n}\right)^{-\hat{\alpha}} - \left(\frac{n_i}{n}\right)^{-\hat{\alpha}} \right\} \right]^{-1/\hat{\alpha}},$$

where $n_i = \sum_{j=1}^{n} \mathbf{I}(t_j \geq t_i)$ is the number at-risk at time t_i. We computed the CG estimator by using the *compound.Cox* R package (Emura et al. 2018).

The separation of the two curves in Fig. 5.3 is measured by the average vertical difference between the survival curves over the *study period*. This statistic is considered as a scaled version of the area between the two survival curves. It is also equivalent to a special case of the weighted Kaplan–Meier statistics (Pepe and Fleming 1989). When using this statistic, the choice of the study period strongly influences the test results. The common choice is the period where at least one survivor exists in both groups (Chap. 2; Klein and Moeschberger 2003). The study period is depicted in Fig. 5.3.

The P-value for testing the difference between the two groups is obtained using the permutation test (Frankel et al. 2007). In each permutation, good prognosis group ($n = 31$) and poor prognosis group ($n = 31$) are randomly allocated from the 62 testing samples, and then, the CG estimator is computed for each group. For each permutation, the study period is determined and the average vertical difference between the two CG estimators is calculated. The P-value is computed as the proportion of 10,000 permuted test statistics exceeding the original test statistic.

The two curves are significantly separated between the good and poor prognoses (Average difference = 0.224; P-value = 0.021). This result justifies the predictive ability of the PI derived by using the copula-based approach.

5.7 Discussions

We have introduced copula-based approaches for selecting genes and making survival prediction in the presence of dependent censoring. The method can be flexibly applied to accommodate different copulas, such as the Clayton, Gumbel, and FGM copulas. Due to its mathematical simplicity, we prefer the Clayton copula to other copulas in modeling dependence structure between survival time and censoring time. However, the effect of dependent censoring on estimates can be remarkably different between different copulas (Chap. 3). Rivest and Wells (2001) theoretically explored the sensitivity of using different copulas on estimating a marginal survival function.

Due to the inherent problem of the non-identifiability of competing risks data (Tsiatis 1975), it is not easy to identify the degree of dependence (i.e., the true copula parameter) between survival and censoring times. The problem is due to the fact that the likelihood function contains little information to identify the true copula parameter. Alternatively, we choose the copula parameter by using a cross-validated *c*-index, a predictive measure free from the likelihood criterion. This method exhibited sound numerical performances in our numerical analyses. Unfortunately, we do not have a theoretical justification of the method, such as consistency. Recently, Emura and Michimae (2017) proposed a goodness-of-fit procedure to test the assumption of the correct copula under competing risks. According to their simulation results, their approaches have certain ability to identify the correct copula under a large number of samples. However, their approaches have not been extended to include covariates.

After relevant genes are selected, researchers often use them to stratify patients between good and poor prognosis groups in validation samples. This is a common strategy to assess prediction performance of the selected genes. Researchers typically use the log-rank test to see how well the Kaplan–Meier survival curves are separated between the good and poor groups. Note that these commonly used validation strategies may give biased results if dependent censoring exists in validation samples. Copulas are used to adjust for this bias by replacing the Kaplan–Meier estimator by the copula-graphic estimator. Since the log-rank test is no longer valid in the presence of dependent censoring, we apply the permutation test based on the average vertical difference between the copula-graphic estimators. For purpose of constructing survival forests, Moradian et al. (2017) also suggested the copula-graphic estimator to measure the difference between two groups under dependent censoring.

One potential drawback of the proposed gene selection method is that it needs to impose a proportional hazards model for the censoring distribution in Eq. (5.3). On the other hand, the traditional univariate Cox regression does not require any model assumption on the censoring distribution. This elimination of the model assumption is the consequence of the independent censoring assumption. Once the independent censoring assumption is relaxed, certain model specifications for the censoring distribution appear to be mandatory (e.g., Siannis et al. 2005; Chen 2010). If the research interest lies in the effect of genes on both survival time and censoring time, the proportional hazards model for the censoring distribution may provide useful information. For instance, researchers may be interested in selecting genes associated with both disease-specific survival and time-to-death due to other causes as in the competing risks setting (Escarela and Carrière 2003).

References

Alizadeh AA, Gentles AJ, Alencar AJ, Liu CL, Kohrt HE et al (2011) Prediction of survival in diffuse large B-cell lymphoma based on the expression of 2 genes reflecting tumor and microenvironment. Blood 118(5):1350–1358

Beer DG, Kardia SLR, Huang CC, Giordano TJ, Levin AM et al (2002) Gene-expression profiles predict survival of patients with lung adenocarcinoma. Nat Med 8:816–824

Bøvelstad HM, Nygård S, Storvold HL, Aldrin M, Borgan Ø et al (2007) Predicting survival from microarray data—a comparative study. Bioinformatics 23:2080–2087

Bøvelstad HM, Nygård S, Borgan Ø (2009) Survival prediction from clinico-genomic models-a comparative study. BMC Bioinf 10(1):1

Chen YH (2010) Semiparametric marginal regression analysis for dependent competing risks under an assumed copula. J R Stat Soc Ser B Stat Methodol 72:235–251

Chen HY, Yu SL, Chen CH, Chang GC, Chen CY et al (2007) A five-gene signature and clinical outcome in non-small-cell lung cancer. N Engl J Med 356:11–20

Emura T, Chen YH, Chen HY (2012). Survival prediction based on compound covariate under Cox proportional hazard models. PLoS One 7(10): e47627, https://doi.org/10.1371/journal.pone.0047627

Emura T, Chen HY, Matsui S, Chen YH (2018). compound.Cox: univariate feature selection and compound covariate for predicting survival, CRAN

Emura T, Chen YH (2016) Gene selection for survival data under dependent censoring, a copula-based approach. Stat Methods Med Res 25(6):2840–2857

Emura T, Michimae H (2017) A copula-based inference to piecewise exponential models under dependent censoring, with application to time to metamorphosis of salamander larvae. Environ Ecol Stat 24(1):151–173

Emura T, Nakatochi M, Matsui S, Michimae H, Rondeau V (2017) Personalized dynamic prediction of death according to tumour progression and high-dimensional genetic factors: meta-analysis with a joint model. Stat Methods Med Res, https://doi.org/10.1177/0962280216688032

Escarela G, Carrière JF (2003) Fitting competing risks with an assumed copula. Stat Methods Med Res 12(4):333–349

Frankel PH, Reid ME, Marshall JR (2007) A permutation test for a weighted Kaplan-Meier estimator with application to the nutritional prevention of cancer trial. Contemp Clin Trial 28:343–347

Harrell FE, Califf RM, Pryor DB, Lee KL, Rosati RA (1982) Evaluating the yield of medical tests. JAMA 247:2543–2546

Hastie T, Tibshirani R, Friedman J (2009) The elements of statistical learning. Springer, New York

Jenssen TK, Kuo WP, Stokke T, Hovig E (2002) Association between gene expressions in breast cancer and patient survival. Hum Genet 111:411–420

Klein JP, Moeschberger ML (2003) Survival analysis techniques for censored and truncated data. Springer, New York

Lossos IS, Czerwinski DK, Alizadeh AA, Wechser MA, Tibshirani R, Botstein D, Levy R (2004) Prediction of survival in diffuse large-B-cell lymphoma based on the expression of six genes. N Engl J Med 350(18):1828–1837

Matsui S (2006) Predicting survival outcomes using subsets of significant genes in prognostic marker studies with microarrays. BMC Bioinf 7:156

Matsui S, Simon RM, Qu P, Shaughnessy JD, Barlogie B, Crowley J (2012) Developing and validating continuous genomic signatures in randomized clinical trials for predictive medicine. Clin Cancer Res 18(21):6065–6073

Michiels S, Koscielny S, Hill C (2005) Prediction of cancer outcome with microarrays: a multiple random validation strategy. Lancet 365(9458):488–492

Moradian H, Denis Larocque D, Bellavance F (2017). Survival forests for data with dependent censoring. Stat Methods Med Res, https://doi.org/10.1177/0962280217727314

Nelsen RB (2006) An introduction to copulas, 2nd edn. Springer, New York

Pepe MS, Fleming TR (1989). Weighted Kaplan-Meier statistics: a class of distance tests for censored survival data. Biometrics: 497–507

Popple A, Durrant LG, Spendlove I, Scott PRI, Deen S, Ramage JM (2012) The chemokine, CXCL12, is an independent predictor of poor survival in ovarian cancer. Br J Cancer 106:1306–1313

Rivest LP, Wells MT (2001) A martingale approach to the copula-graphic estimator for the survival function under dependent censoring. J Multivar Anal 79:138–155

Sabatier R, Finetti P, Adelaide J, Guille A, Borg JP, Chaffanet M, Bertucci F (2011) Down-regulation of ECRG4, a candidate tumor suppressor gene, in human breast cancer. PLoS One 6(11):e27656

Schumacher M, Binder H, Gerds T (2007) Assessment of survival prediction models based on microarray data. Bioinformatics 23(14):1768–1774

Shedden K, Taylor JMG, Enkemann SA, Tsao MS, Yeatman TJ et al (2008) Gene expression-based survival prediction in lung adenocarcinoma: a multi-site, blinded validation study. Nat Med 14:822–827

Siannis F, Copas J, Lu G (2005) Sensitivity analysis for informative censoring in parametric survival models. Biostatistics 6(1):77–91

Sklar A (1959) Fonctions de répartition à n dimensions et leurs marges. Publications de l'Institut de Statistique de L'Université de Paris. 8:229–31

Tsiatis A (1975) A nonidentifiability aspect of the problem of competing risks. Proc Natl Acad Sci 72(1):20–22

Tukey JW (1993) Tightening the clinical trial. Control Clin Trials 14:266–285

Yoshihara K, Tajima A, Yahata T, Kodama S, Fujiwara H et al (2010) Gene expression profile for predicting survival in advanced-stage serous ovarian cancer across two independent datasets. PLoS One 5(3):e9615

Yoshihara K, Tsunoda T, Shigemizu D, Fujiwara H, Hatae M et al (2012) High-risk ovarian cancer based on 126-gene expression signature is uniquely characterized by downregulation of antigen presentation pathway. Clin Cancer Res 18(5):1374–1385

van Wieringen WN, Kun D, Hampel R, Boulesteix AL (2009) Survival prediction using gene expression data: a review and comparison. Comput Stat Data Anal 53(5):1590–1603

Verveij PJM, van Houwelingen HC (1993) Crossvalidation in survival analysis. Stat Med 12:2305–2314

Waldron L, Haibe-Kains B, Culhane AC, Riester M, Ding J et al. (2014) Comparative meta-analysis of prognostic gene signatures for late-stage ovarian cancer. J Natl Cancer Inst 106(5): dju049

Wang Y, Klijn JG, Zhang Y, Sieuwerts AM et al (2005) Gene-expression profiles to predict distant metastasis of lymph-node-negative primary breast cancer. Lancet 365(9460):671–679

Witten DM, Tibshirani R (2010) Survival analysis with high-dimensional covariates. Stat Methods Med Res 19(1):29–51

Zhao X, Rødland EA, Sørlie T, Naume B, Langerød A et al (2011) Combining gene signatures improves prediction of breast cancer survival. PLoS One 6(3):e17845

Zhao SD, Parmigiani G, Huttenhower C, Waldron L (2014) Más-o-menos: a simple sign averaging method for discrimination in genomic data analysis. Bioinformatics 30(21):3062–3069

Chapter 6
Future Developments

Abstract This final chapter introduces two open problems for future research. This might help find research topics for students and researchers.

Keywords Copula-graphic estimator · Dependent truncation · Left-truncation Log-rank test

6.1 Log-Rank Test Under Dependent Censoring

The three most important statistical methods in survival analysis would be the Kaplan–Meier estimator, the log-rank test, and Cox regression. These three methods adopt simple ways to deal with censoring. However, these methods critically rely on the validity of the independent censoring assumption (Chap. 2).

The copula-graphic estimator (Zheng and Klein 1995; Rivest and Wells 2001) is a natural generalization of the Kaplan–Meier estimator in the presence of dependent censoring. Also, the semi-parametric maximum likelihood estimator of Chen (2010) is a natural generalization of Cox regression (Chap. 4). These methods for dependent censoring utilize copulas to adjust for the effect of dependent censoring, and they reduce to the original methods under the independence copula. However, the copula-based generalization of the log-rank test under dependent censoring has not been considered in the literature.

Researchers often wish to separate patients between good and poor prognosis groups and then use the log-rank test to see how well the Kaplan–Meier survival curves are separated between the good and poor groups. This strategy may give biased results if dependent censoring exists in the samples (Emura and Chen 2016; Moradian et al. 2017). In Chap. 5, we apply a permutation test based on the difference between the two survival curves calculated by the copula-graphic estimator. While this approach can account for the effect of dependent censoring, it is not regarded as the log-rank test. The log-rank test should compare the hazard rates between two groups rather than the survival curves.

© The Author(s) 2018

T. Emura and Y.-H. Chen, *Analysis of Survival Data with Dependent Censoring*, JSS Research Series in Statistics, https://doi.org/10.1007/978-981-10-7164-5_6

Hence, it is interesting to develop an alternative two-sample test, similar to the log-rank test, under dependent censoring. In general, two copulas are necessary for two groups (e.g., good and poor prognosis groups). A starting point may be the assumption that the copula is the same in the two groups, as we have assumed in Chap. 5. While deriving a generalized log-rank test under an assumed copula, it is relevant to study the robustness or sensitivity of the test against copula misspecification as in Rivest and Wells (2001). Based on the sensitivity analysis of Chap. 3, we conjecture that the log-rank test is robust against the effect of dependent censoring modeled via the Gumbel copula.

6.2 Dependent Left-Truncation

Left-truncation often occurs if survival time is measured from birth. In this case, survival analysis may be based on the age-specific hazard function and left-truncation time corresponds to entry age (should not be treated as covariates). This book does not discuss the problem of left-truncation since the theme is focused on censoring. Meanwhile, it is of great interest to design aging research under left-truncation (e.g., Rodríguez-Girondo et al. 2016), where the issue of *dependent* left-truncation may arise in addition to the issue of dependent censoring.

Traditional analyses for left-truncated survival data rely on the *independent truncation* assumption (p.126 of Klein and Moeschberger 2003). For instance, in survival analysis of elderly residents, the age at entry to a retirement center is assumed to be independent of age at death (Hyde 1980). Several different tests for checking the assumption of independent truncation were developed (Emura and Wang 2010). The effect of dependent truncation in competing risks analysis was studied by Bakoyannis and Touloumi (2017). To fit survival data with dependent left-truncation, a copula model between event time and left-truncation time has been considered (Chaieb et al. 2006; Emura and Wang 2012; Emura and Murotani 2015; Emura and Pan 2017). However, these methods cannot be directly applied to the case where event time is subject to both dependent censoring and dependent truncation. In this case, one may consider two copulas, one for dependent truncation and the other for dependent censoring. One may also consider a copula for dependence between truncation time and censoring time.

References

Bakoyannis G, Touloumi G (2017) Impact of dependent left truncation in semiparametric competing risks methods: a simulation study. Commun Stat Simul Comput 46(3):2025–2042
Chaieb LL, Rivest LP, Abdous B (2006) Estimating survival under a dependent truncation. Biometrika 93(3):655–669
Chen YH (2010) Semiparametric marginal regression analysis for dependent competing risks under an assumed copula. J R Stat Soc Ser B Stat Methodol 72:235–251

Emura T, Chen YH (2016) Gene selection for survival data under dependent censoring, a copula-based approach. Stat Methods Med Res 25(6):2840–2857

Emura T, Murotani K (2015) An algorithm for estimating survival under a copula-based dependent truncation model. Test 24(4):734–751

Emura T, Pan CH (2017) Parametric likelihood inference and goodness-of-fit for dependently left-truncated data, a copula-based approach, Stat Pap, https://doi.org/10.1007/s00362-017-0947-z

Emura T, Wang W (2010) Testing quasi-independence for truncation data. J Multivar Anal 101:223–239

Emura T, Wang W (2012) Nonparametric maximum likelihood estimation for dependent truncation data based on copulas. J Multivar Anal 110:171–188

Hyde J (1980) Survival analysis with incomplete observations. In: Miller RG, Efron B, Brown BW, Moses LE (eds) Biostatistics casebook. Wiley, New York, pp 31–46

Klein JP, Moeschberger ML (2003) Survival analysis techniques for censored and truncated data. Springer, New York

Moradian H, Denis Larocque D, Bellavance F (2017). Survival forests for data with dependent censoring, Stat Methods Med Res, https://doi.org/10.1177/0962280217727314

Rivest LP, Wells MT (2001) A martingale approach to the copula-graphic estimator for the survival function under dependent censoring. J Multivar Anal 79:138–155

Rodríguez-Girondo M, Deelen J, Slagboom EP, Houwing-Duistermaat JJ (2016). Survival analysis with delayed entry in selected families with application to human longevity. Stat Methods Med Res, https://doi.org/10.1177/0962280216648356

Zheng M, Klein JP (1995) Estimates of marginal survival for dependent competing risks based on an assumed copula. Biometrika 82(1):127–138

Appendix A
Spline Basis Functions

This appendix defines the spline basis functions used in $\lambda_0(t) = \sum_{\ell=1}^{5} g_\ell M_\ell(t) = \mathbf{g}'\mathbf{M}(t)$. We then explain how $M_\ell(t)$'s are derived. We also calculate the roughness $\int \ddot{\lambda}_0(t)^2 dt$.

For a knot sequence $\xi_1 < \xi_2 < \xi_3$ with an equally spaced mesh $\Delta = \xi_2 - \xi_1 = \xi_3 - \xi_2$, let $z_i(t) = (t - \xi_i)/\Delta$ for $i = 1, 2$, and 3. Define *M-spline basis* functions

$$M_1(t) = -\frac{4\mathbf{I}(\xi_1 \le t < \xi_2)}{\Delta} z_2(t)^3, \quad M_5(t) = \frac{4\mathbf{I}(\xi_2 \le t < \xi_3)}{\Delta} z_2(t)^3,$$

$$M_2(t) = \frac{\mathbf{I}(\xi_1 \le t < \xi_2)}{2\Delta}\{7z_1(t)^3 - 18z_1(t)^2 + 12z_1(t)\} - \frac{\mathbf{I}(\xi_2 \le t < \xi_3)}{2\Delta} z_3(t)^3,$$

$$M_3(t) = \frac{\mathbf{I}(\xi_1 \le t < \xi_2)}{\Delta}\{-2z_1(t)^3 + 3z_1(t)^2\} + \frac{\mathbf{I}(\xi_2 \le t < \xi_3)}{\Delta}\{2z_2(t)^3 - 3z_2(t)^2 + 1\},$$

$$M_4(t) = \frac{\mathbf{I}(\xi_1 \le t < \xi_2)}{2\Delta} z_1(t)^3 + \frac{\mathbf{I}(\xi_2 \le t < \xi_3)}{2\Delta}\{-7z_2(t)^3 + 3z_2(t)^2 + 3z_2(t) + 1\}.$$

Define the *I-spline basis* function, $I_\ell(t) = \int_{\xi_1}^{t} M_\ell(u)du$, which can be written as

$$I_1(t) = 1 - z_2(t)^4 \mathbf{I}(\xi_1 \le t < \xi_2), \quad I_5(t) = z_2(t)^4 \mathbf{I}(\xi_2 \le t < \xi_3),$$

$$I_2(t) = \left\{\frac{7}{8}z_1(t)^4 - 3z_1(t)^3 + 3z_1(t)^2\right\}\mathbf{I}(\xi_1 \le t < \xi_2) + \left\{1 - \frac{1}{8}z_3(t)^4\right\}\mathbf{I}(\xi_2 \le t < \xi_3),$$

$$I_3(t) = \left\{-\frac{1}{2}z_1(t)^4 + z_1(t)^3\right\}\mathbf{I}(\xi_1 \le t < \xi_2) + \left\{\frac{1}{2} + \frac{1}{2}z_2(t)^4 - z_2(t)^3 + z_2(t)\right\}\mathbf{I}(\xi_2 \le t < \xi_3),$$

$$I_4(t) = \frac{1}{8}z_1(t)^4 \mathbf{I}(\xi_1 \le t < \xi_2) + \left\{\frac{1}{8} - \frac{7}{8}z_2(t)^4 + \frac{1}{2}z_2(t)^3 + \frac{3}{4}z_2(t)^2 + \frac{1}{2}z_2(t)\right\}\mathbf{I}(\xi_2 \le t < \xi_3).$$

© The Author(s) 2018

T. Emura and Y.-H. Chen, *Analysis of Survival Data with Dependent Censoring*,
JSS Research Series in Statistics, https://doi.org/10.1007/978-981-10-7164-5

The second derivatives of the M-spline basis functions are

$$\ddot{M}_1(t) = -\frac{24}{\Delta^3} z_2(t) \mathbf{I}(\xi_1 \le t < \xi_2), \quad \ddot{M}_5(t) = \frac{24}{\Delta^3} z_2(t) \mathbf{I}(\xi_2 \le t < \xi_3),$$

$$\ddot{M}_2(t) = \left\{ \frac{21}{\Delta^3} z_1(t) - \frac{18}{\Delta^3} \right\} \mathbf{I}(\xi_1 \le t < \xi_2) - \frac{3}{\Delta^3} z_3(t) \mathbf{I}(\xi_2 \le t < \xi_3),$$

$$\ddot{M}_3(t) = \left\{ -\frac{12}{\Delta^3} z_1(t) + \frac{6}{\Delta^3} \right\} \mathbf{I}(\xi_1 \le t < \xi_2) + \left\{ \frac{12}{\Delta^3} z_2(t) - \frac{6}{\Delta^3} \right\} \mathbf{I}(\xi_2 \le t < \xi_3),$$

$$\ddot{M}_4(t) = \frac{3}{\Delta^3} z_1(t) \mathbf{I}(\xi_1 \le t < \xi_2) + \left\{ -\frac{21}{\Delta^3} z_2(t) + \frac{3}{\Delta^3} \right\} \mathbf{I}(\xi_2 \le t < \xi_3).$$

It follows that

$$\int \ddot{M}_1(t)^2 dt = \frac{192}{\Delta^5}, \int \ddot{M}_2(t)^2 dt = \frac{96}{\Delta^5}, \int \ddot{M}_3(t)^2 dt = \frac{24}{\Delta^5}, \int \ddot{M}_4(t)^2 dt = \frac{96}{\Delta^5}, \int \ddot{M}_5(t)^2 dt = \frac{192}{\Delta^5},$$

$$\int \ddot{M}_1(t)\ddot{M}_2(t) dt = -\frac{132}{\Delta^5}, \int \ddot{M}_1(t)\ddot{M}_3(t) dt = \frac{24}{\Delta^5}, \int \ddot{M}_1(t)\ddot{M}_4(t) dt = \frac{12}{\Delta^5}, \int \ddot{M}_1(t)\ddot{M}_5(t) dt = 0,$$

$$\int \ddot{M}_2(t)\ddot{M}_3(t) dt = -\frac{24}{\Delta^5}, \int \ddot{M}_2(t)\ddot{M}_4(t) dt = -\frac{12}{\Delta^5}, \int \ddot{M}_2(t)\ddot{M}_5(t) dt = \frac{12}{\Delta^5},$$

$$\int \ddot{M}_3(t)\ddot{M}_4(t) dt = -\frac{24}{\Delta^5}, \int \ddot{M}_3(t)\ddot{M}_5(t) dt = \frac{24}{\Delta^5}, \int \ddot{M}_4(t)\ddot{M}_5(t) dt = -\frac{132}{\Delta^5},$$

where the range of integral is $(\xi_1, \xi_3]$. Then, the penalization term is explicitly computed as

$$\int \ddot{\lambda}_0(t)^2 dt = \sum_{k=1}^{5} \sum_{\ell=1}^{5} g_k g_\ell \int \ddot{M}_k(t) \ddot{M}_\ell(t) dt$$

$$= \frac{1}{\Delta^5} \mathbf{g}' \begin{bmatrix} 192 & -132 & 24 & 12 & 0 \\ -132 & 96 & -24 & -12 & 12 \\ 24 & -24 & 24 & -24 & 24 \\ 12 & -12 & -24 & 96 & -132 \\ 0 & 12 & 24 & -132 & 192 \end{bmatrix} \mathbf{g} = \mathbf{g}' \Omega \mathbf{g}.$$

All the expressions mentioned above were derived in the supplementary material of Emura et al. (2017). The computational programs of the M- and I-spline basis functions are available in the *joint.Cox* R package (Emura 2018). These basis functions were derived from the general definition of M-spline basis functions given by Ramsay (1988). Below, we shall explain the details about the derivations.

The M-spline basis functions are defined on an interval $[L, U]$ which is subdivided by a knot sequence $L = \xi_1 < \cdots < \xi_q = U$. We set another knot sequence

$t_1 \leq t_2 \cdots \leq t_{n+k}$ such that $t_1 = \cdots = t_k = L$ and $t_{n+1} = \cdots = t_{n+k} = U$. Then, the M-spline bases of degree $k - 1$ are recursively defined as:

For $k = 1$

$$M_i(t|k = 1) = \frac{1}{t_{i+1} - t_i} \quad if \quad t_i \leq t < t_{i+1},$$

$$M_i(t|k = 1) = 0 \qquad otherwise.$$

For $k > 1$,

$$M_i(t|k) = \frac{k\{(t - t_i)M_i(t|k - 1) + (t_{i+k} - t)M_{i+1}(t|k - 1)\}}{(k - 1)(t_{i+k} - t_i)}.$$

The cubic spline bases correspond to $k = 4$, giving cubic polynomials in t. Our derivations are based on $t_1 = \cdots = t_4 = \xi_1$, $t_5 = \xi_2$, and $t_6 = \cdots = t_9 = \xi_3$ with the equally spaced mesh $\Delta = \xi_2 - \xi_1 = \xi_3 - \xi_2$. In the following, we provide the detailed derivations of some functions.

- **Derivation of** $M_1(t) = -\frac{4I(\xi_1 \leq t < \xi_2)}{\Delta} z_2(t)^3$.

We derive $M_1(t|k = 4)$ in knot intervals of $[t_4 \leq t < t_5]$. Then, the M-spline basis functions are recursively computed as

$M_4(t|k = 1) = \frac{1}{\Delta}$,

$M_3(t|k = 1) = 0$,

$M_3(t|k = 2) = \frac{2\{(t - t_3)M_3(t|k = 1) + (t_5 - t)M_4(t|k = 1)\}}{(2 - 1)\Delta} = \frac{2(t_5 - t)}{\Delta^2}$,

$M_2(t|k = 2) = 0$,

$M_2(t|k = 3) = \frac{3\{(t - t_2)M_2(t|k = 2) + (t_5 - t)M_3(t|k = 2)\}}{(3 - 1)\Delta} = \frac{3(t_5 - t)}{2\Delta} \cdot \frac{2(t_5 - t)}{\Delta^2} = \frac{3(t_5 - t)^2}{\Delta^3}$,

$M_1(t|k = 3) = 0$,

$M_1(t|k = 4) = \frac{4\{(t - t_1)M_1(t|k = 3) + (t_5 - t)M_2(t|k = 3)\}}{(4 - 1)\Delta} = \frac{4(t_5 - t)}{3\Delta} \cdot \frac{3(t_5 - t)^2}{\Delta^3} = -\frac{4}{\Delta}z_2(t)^3$,

So one can obtain

$$M_1(t|k = 4) = -\frac{4z_2(t)^3}{\Delta}I(\xi_1 \leq t < \xi_2).$$

- **Derivation of** $M_2(t) = \dfrac{I(\xi_1 \le t < \xi_2)}{2\Delta}\{\,7z_1(t)^3 - 18z_1(t)^2 + 12z_1(t)\,\} - \dfrac{I(\xi_2 \le t < \xi_3)}{2\Delta}\,z_3(t)^3$

We shall derive $M_2(t|k=4)$ in the interval $[t_4 \le t < t_5]$ and interval $[t_5 \le t < t_6]$, separately. First, we derive $M_2(t|k=4)$ in $[t_4 \le t < t_5]$. By the definition,

$$M_5(t|k=1) = 0$$

$$M_4(t|k=2) = \frac{2\{(t-t_4)M_4(t|k=1) + (t_6-t)M_5(t|k=1)\}}{(2-1)(t_6-t_4)} = \frac{(t-t_4)}{\Delta^2}$$

$$M_3(t|k=3) = \frac{3\{(t-t_3)M_3(t|k=2) + (t_6-t)M_4(t|k=2)\}}{(3-1)(t_6-t_3)}$$

$$= \frac{3}{2(2\Delta)}\left\{\frac{2(t-t_3)(t_5-t)}{\Delta^2} + \frac{(t_6-t)(t-t_4)}{\Delta^2}\right\}$$

$$= \frac{3\{2(t-\xi_1)(\xi_2-t) + (\xi_3-t)(t-\xi_1)\}}{4\Delta^3}$$

$$= -\frac{3}{4\Delta}\{2z_1(t)z_2(t) + z_1(t)z_3(t)\},$$

$$M_2(t|k=4) = \frac{4\{(t-t_2)M_2(t|k=3) + (t_6-t)M_3(t|k=3)\}}{(4-1)(t_6-t_2)}$$

$$= \frac{4}{3(2\Delta)}\left[\frac{3(t-t_2)(t_5-t)^2}{\Delta^3} + \frac{-3(t_6-t)\{2z_1(t)z_2(t) + z_1(t)z_3(t)\}}{4\Delta}\right]$$

$$= \frac{1}{2\Delta}\left[\frac{4(t-\xi_1)(\xi_2-t)^2}{\Delta^3} + \frac{-(\xi_3-t)\{2z_1(t)z_2(t) + z_1(t)z_3(t)\}}{\Delta}\right]$$

$$= \frac{1}{2\Delta}\left[4z_1(t)z_2(t)^2 + z_3\{2z_1(t)z_2(t) + z_1(t)z_3(t)\}\right].$$

Note that $\xi_2 = \Delta + \xi_1$ and $\xi_3 = 2\Delta + \xi_1$. So $z_2(t)$ and $z_3(t)$ are derived as $z_2(t) = z_1(t) - 1$ and $z_3(t) = z_1(t) - 2$, respectively. Then, one can obtain $M_2(t|k=4)$ in $[t_4 \le t < t_5]$ as follows.

$$M_2(t|k=4) = \frac{1}{2\Delta}\left\{7z_1(t)^3 - 18z_1(t)^2 + 12z_1(t)\right\}I(\xi_1 \le t < \xi_2).$$

Next, we derive $M_2(t|k=4)$ in $[t_5 \le t < t_6]$. It follows that

$$M_5(t|k=1) = \frac{1}{\Delta},$$

$$M_4(t|k=1) = 0,$$

$$M_4(t|k=2) = \frac{2\{(t-t_4)M_4(t|k=1) + (t_6-t)M_5(t|k=1)\}}{(2-1)(t_6-t_4)} = \frac{(t_6-t)}{\Delta^2},$$

$$M_3(t|k=2) = 0,$$

$$M_3(t|k=3) = \frac{3\{(t-t_3)M_3(t|k=2) + (t_6-t)M_4(t|k=2)\}}{(3-1)(t_6-t_3)} = \frac{3(t_6-t)^2}{4\Delta^3},$$

$$M_2(t|k=3) = 0,$$

$$M_2(t|k=4) = \frac{4\{(t-t_2)M_2(t|k=3) + (t_6-t)M_3(t|k=3)\}}{(4-1)(t_6-t_2)}$$

$$= \frac{(t_6-t)^3}{2\Delta^4} = -\frac{z_3(t)^3}{2\Delta}.$$

So one can obtain $M_2(t|k=4)$ in $[t_5 \leq t < t_6]$ as

$$M_2(t|k=4) = -\frac{z_3(t)^3}{2\Delta}I(\xi_2 \leq t < \xi_3).$$

Combining the two cases for $M_2(t|k=4)$, one can obtain the desired result as

$$M_2(t|k=4) = \frac{1}{2\Delta}\left\{7z_1(t)^3 - 18z_1(t)^2 + 12z_1(t)\right\}I(\xi_1 \leq t < \xi_2)$$

$$- \frac{z_3(t)^3}{2\Delta}I(\xi_2 \leq t < \xi_3).$$

- **Derivation of** $\int \ddot{M}_1(t)^2 dt = \frac{192}{\Delta^5}$ **and** $\int \ddot{M}_1(t)\ddot{M}_2(t)dt = -\frac{132}{\Delta^5}$

The derivatives of the M-spline basis functions are

$$\dot{M}_1(t|k=4) = -\frac{12I(\xi_1 \leq t < \xi_2)}{\Delta^2}z_2(t)^2,$$

$$\ddot{M}_1(t|k=4) = -\frac{24I(\xi_1 \leq t < \xi_2)}{\Delta^3}z_2(t),$$

$$\dot{M}_2(t|k=4) = \frac{1}{2\Delta^2}\left\{21z_1(t)^2 - 36z_1(t) + 12\right\}I(\xi_1 \leq t < \xi_2) - \frac{3z_3(t)^2}{2\Delta^2}I(\xi_2 \leq t < \xi_3),$$

$$\ddot{M}_2(t|k=4) = \left\{\frac{21z_1(t)}{\Delta^3} - \frac{18}{\Delta^3}\right\}I(\xi_1 \leq t < \xi_2) - \frac{3z_3(t)}{\Delta^3}I(\xi_2 \leq t < \xi_3).$$

By integrating $\ddot{M}_1(t|k=4)^2$ on the interval $(\xi_1, \xi_3]$,

$$\int \ddot{M}_1(t)^2 dt = \int \frac{(-24)^2}{\Delta^6} \cdot \frac{(t-\xi_2)^2}{\Delta^2} I(\xi_1 \leq t < \xi_2) dt = \frac{576}{\Delta^8} \int (t-\xi_2)^2 I(\xi_1 \leq t < \xi_2) dt$$

$$= \frac{576}{\Delta^8} \left[\frac{(t-\xi_2)^3}{3} I(\xi_1 \leq t < \xi_2) \right]_{t-\xi_1}^{\xi_2} = \frac{576}{\Delta^8} \left\{ 0 - \frac{(-\Delta)^3}{3} \right\} = \frac{192}{\Delta^5}.$$

By integrating $\ddot{M}_1(t)\ddot{M}_2(t)$ on the interval $(\xi_1, \xi_3]$,

$$\int \ddot{M}_1(t)\ddot{M}_2(t) dt = \int -\frac{24z_2(t)I(\xi_1 \leq t < \xi_2)}{\Delta^3} \left[\left\{ \frac{21}{\Delta^3} z_1(t) - \frac{18}{\Delta^3} \right\} I(\xi_1 \leq t < \xi_2) - \frac{3}{\Delta^3} z_3(t) I(\xi_2 \leq t < \xi_3) \right] dt$$

The product of $I(\xi_1 \leq t < \xi_2)$ and $I(\xi_2 \leq t < \xi_3)$ is equal to 0. Hence,

$$\int \ddot{M}_1(t)\ddot{M}_2(t) dt = \int -\frac{24z_2(t)I(\xi_1 \leq t < \xi_2)}{\Delta^3} \cdot \left\{ \frac{21}{\Delta^3} z_1(t) - \frac{18}{\Delta^3} \right\} I(\xi_1 \leq t < \xi_2) dt$$

$$= \int -\frac{504}{\Delta^8}(\Delta + t - \xi_2)(t - \xi_2) I(\xi_1 \leq t < \xi_2) + \frac{432}{\Delta^7}(\Delta + t - \xi_2) I(\xi_1 \leq t < \xi_2) dt$$

$$= -\frac{504}{\Delta^8} \left[\frac{1}{3}(t - \xi_2)^3 + \frac{1}{2}\Delta(t - \xi_2)^2 \right]_{t-\xi_1}^{\xi_2} I(\xi_1 \leq t < \xi_2) + \frac{432}{\Delta^7} \left[\frac{1}{2}\Delta(t - \varepsilon_2)^2 \right]_{t-\xi_1}^{\xi_2} I(\xi_1 \leq t < \xi_2)$$

$$= -\frac{504}{\Delta^8} \left\{ \frac{-1}{3}(-\Delta)^3 - \frac{1}{2}\Delta^3 \right\} + \frac{432}{\Delta^7} \left(-\frac{1}{2}\Delta^2 \right) = \frac{84}{\Delta^5} - \frac{216}{\Delta^5} = -\frac{132}{\Delta^5}.$$

References

Emura T, Nakatochi M, Murotani K, Rondeau V (2017). A joint frailty-copula model between tumour progression and death for meta-analysis, Stat Methods Med Res 26 (6): 2649–2666.

Emura T (2018). joint.Cox: penalized likelihood estimation and dynamic prediction under the joint frailty-copula models between tumour progression and death for meta-analysis, CRAN

Ramsay J (1988). Monotone regression spline in action. Statis Sci 3:425–61.

Appendix B
R Codes for the Lung Cancer Data Analysis

```
library(compound.Cox)
data(Lung) # read the data
temp=Lung[,"train"] # indicators for training/testing samples #
t.vec=Lung[temp,"t.vec"] # death or censoring times for 63 training samples #
d.vec=Lung[temp,"d.vec"] # censoring indicators for 63 training samples #
X.mat=as.matrix( Lung[temp,-c(1,2,3)] ) # a matrix of gene expressions (63 by 97 elements) #

res=dependCox.reg.CV(t.vec,d.vec,X.mat,K=5,G=20) # fit Cox regression models
res

Beta=res$beta
P=res$P
###### Outputs sorted by P-values #######
cbind(Coef=round(Beta[order(P)],2),P.value=round(sort(P),4))

####### Prediction accuracy for testing data #######
alpha=res$alpha
temp_te=Lung[,"train"]==FALSE
t.vec=Lung[temp_te,"t.vec"]
d.vec=Lung[temp_te,"d.vec"]
X.mat=Lung[temp_te,-c(1,2,3)]
n=nrow(X.mat)
```

© The Author(s) 2018

T. Emura and Y.-H. Chen, *Analysis of Survival Data with Dependent Censoring*,
JSS Research Series in Statistics, https://doi.org/10.1007/978-981-10-7164-5

```
temp_P=P<=sort(P)[16]  ## Top 16 genes ##
PI=as.matrix(X.mat[,temp_P])%*%Beta[temp_P]
t.oeta=t.vec[order(PI)]
d.oeta=d.vec[order(PI)]

###### Plot the CG estimators #####
temp=1:floor(n/2)
t.good=t.oeta[temp]
d.good=d.oeta[temp]
S.good=CG.Clayton(t.good,d.good,alpha,S.plot=TRUE,S.col="blue")$surv

t.poor=t.oeta[-temp]
d.poor=d.oeta[-temp]
S.poor=CG.Clayton(t.poor,d.poor,alpha,S.plot=TRUE,S.col="red")$surv

plot(c(0,sort(t.good)),c(1,S.good),type="s",lwd=3,xlim=c(0,55),ylim=c(0.2,1),
    col="blue",ylab="Survival probability",xlab="Months")
points(sort(t.good[d.good==0]),S.good[d.good[order(t.good)]==0],pch=3,cex=2,col="blue")
points(c(0,sort(t.poor)),c(1,S.poor),type="s",lwd=3,col="red")
points(sort(t.poor[d.poor==0]),S.poor[d.poor[order(t.poor)]==0],pch=3,cex=2,col="red")
```

The codes need 30 minutes to an hour to finish the computation.

Index

T. Emura and Y.-H. Chen, *Analysis of Survival Data with Dependent Censoring*,
JSS Research Series in Statistics, https://doi.org/10.1007/978-981-10-7164-5

Printed in the United States
By Bookmasters